The Amazing Results of
Hormone Replacement Therapy

D1586515

'There were times when I sat in my flat and contemplated suicide, I was so depressed by what was happening to me, but since I started HRT I've been a new woman. I'm no longer nervy, moody and weepy; I've got better skin, more energy and more lust for life than ever before.' *Lynne Perrie*

'I've always looked after myself, eating carefully, taking exercise and so on, and that does help stave off many problems. But ultimately HRT does the most to restore your drive, energy and interest in life, and you stay fit and healthy, instead of being consigned to some scrapyard, old before you need or want to be.' *Adrienne Corri*

'It makes you look better, feel better and generally turns you into the positive, energetic person you were before your hormones let you down. It makes all the difference in the world.' *Jill Gascoine*

The Amarant Book of
Hormone Replacement Therapy

Teresa Gorman MP, a professional biologist and international businesswoman, was at the peak of her career when she was devastated by the effects of the menopause. Fortunately, Doctor Malcolm Whitehead of King's College Hospital prescribed hormone replacement treatment which miraculously restored her vitality and zest for life.

Her experience of the difficulty of getting treatment led her to found the Amarant Trust to redress the ignorance which surrounds this critical event in every woman's life. The Trust also seeks to raise funds for a national research and training centre.

Since 1987, when she was elected to Parliament, she has campaigned for better healthcare for mature women and for the establishment of specialist treatment centres round the country.

Dr Malcolm Whitehead FRCOG is recognized as an international authority on the effects of oestrogen and HRT in women. He is Senior Lecturer in the Academic Department of Obstetrics and Gynaecology of King's College School of Medicine and Dentistry. He is also Honorary Consultant Obstetrician and Gynaecologist to King's College Hospital, which has a worldwide reputation for original research into healthcare for mature women. The menopause unit at King's, which is under Malcolm Whitehead's direction, has been at the forefront of developing newer, safer forms of HRT over the last fifteen years. Many of the HRT preparations currently used by thousands of UK women were developed at King's.

Malcolm Whitehead is also Treasurer of the Executive Committee of the International Menopause Society; a member of the American Fertility Society; and a founder member of the International Society of Gynaecological Endocrinology. He also directs the menopause unit at Queen Charlotte's Maternity Hospital.

'HRT is the greatest treasure of a middle-aged woman's life. I've reached fifty but feel twenty . . .'

These are the words of just one woman whose life has been revolutionized by HRT but they echo those of many thousands of women all over the world who feel the same.

All royalties from the sales of this book will be donated to the Amarant Trust.

The Amarant Book of Hormone Replacement Therapy

How HRT can dramatically reduce all the symptoms connected with the menopause and protect against heart attacks, strokes, osteoporosis, as well as improving memory and concentration

Teresa Gorman MP
and
Dr Malcolm Whitehead

PAN ORIGINAL
PAN BOOKS LONDON, SYDNEY AND AUCKLAND

Acknowledgements

The authors are greatly indebted to Audrey Slaughter, journalist and author, who worked so hard to compile the main structure of this book from interviews with many women on HRT and with medical experts in the field.

They are also grateful to Barbara Cartland and Wendy Cooper who pioneered information on Hormone Replacement Therapy.

First published 1989 by Pan Books Ltd
Cavaye Place, London SW10 9PG
9 8 7 6 5 4 3 2 1
Copyright © The Amarant Trust 1989
ISBN 0 330 31022 4

Photoset by Parker Typesetting Service, Leicester
Printed and bound in Great Britain by
Cox & Wyman Ltd, Reading

Contents

Introduction

WHY THE AMARANT TRUST WAS SET UP

I HAD NOT IMAGINED when I decided to set up the Amarant Trust how much suffering I would uncover, nor how much callous indifference there is towards women who were experiencing the effects of the menopause. Nor did I realize that lives could be redeemed and marriages saved by the application of a simple treatment known as hormone replacement therapy.

My own experience with the menopause had made me determined to help other women by bringing the subject out into the open. The first article I wrote in the *Daily Mail* brought a deluge of letters – 10,000 of them – and the paper had to employ two of its staff for three weeks just to deal with them. Almost every letter was a cry for help. That's when I knew that the Amarant Trust would fill a real need for mature women facing the menopause alone.

For as long as anyone can remember the menopause has been one of those subjects that nobody likes to talk about. Women refer to it in whispers as the 'change of life'. Most men, even married men, can't bear to mention it at all, except to make jokes about it, and usually very unsympathetic ones at that.

It is barely two years since the Amarant Trust was established and already we have brought about a remarkable change in public opinion. We have brought help and hope to thousands of women. And not just women because men, too, are affected by the menopause when their wives or partners take a nose-dive into depression and misery. Now I rarely go to a party without the subject being raised, usually by the man sitting next to me. My male colleagues in the House of Commons attribute my bright appearance and energy at 2 a.m. in the morning to the treatment and ask me if there is anything comparable for them. Recently, I shared a ride from Aberdeen to Edinburgh with four young undergraduates – all men – who wanted to talk about nothing else. One had been asked by his mother to find out as much as possible about the treatment advocated by the Amarant Trust. Another boasted that his mother, after taking hormone replacement therapy, was once more bearable to live with. The third wanted to know for his girlfriend, who would need to know about it – later on.

The menopause – horrid name – is now definitely on the map and a subject of fascination for newspapers, radio and TV, as is hormone replacement therapy or HRT for short. When women reach their mid- to late forties, they begin to lose vital hormones and, as a result, their natural vitality. Suddenly they start to get aches and pains in their joints, hot flushes and depression; they also become forgetful. Life becomes a misery. How can you keep up with a busy domestic life, and maybe a job as well, when you feel as if your body is letting you down?

That's how I felt when the menopause hit me. Fortunately, I had lived in America, where women know all about HRT, and was able to seek treatment. In Britain, however, where most of the pioneering work was done, only about six per cent of women in the relevant age group have access to treatment, despite the fact that it has been available for forty years. There are about nine to ten million women in Britain aged fifty or over, and in any one year approximately 450,000 will experience the menopause. Of these, roughly a third will suffer severe symptoms, but the majority will only be offered tranquillizers or pep pills. Yet medical research shows that replacing the missing hormones can not only give you a trouble-free menopause but help to prevent some of the terrible diseases of old age such as brittle bones, heart attacks and strokes.

By the spring of 1988 the Amarant Trust was receiving over 1,000 letters a week, and interest in the Trust's work was continuing to grow. Within hours of a breakfast TV show with Claire Rayner, for example, we were besieged with calls from women desperate for help. That's when we decided to set up the first Amarant Centre in London, offering counselling and treatment to women who had been refused help locally. It is the prototype for many more centres to come. At present there are only a tiny handful of menopause clinics around the country, hardly any of which are funded by the NHS. This lack of funding means that specialists have to spend time raising money and as a result some clinics in major cities can only afford to open one day a week.

The reason for the lack of clinics is not cruelty or indifference but ignorance. Doctors are not trained in menopause therapy and many still believe that women should put up with symptoms because they are part of the natural process of growing older. But I don't see any point in growing old painfully if it can be avoided. Why shouldn't women enjoy good health in their later years?

Training doctors is therefore another major task for the Amarant Trust. We are raising funds for a national centre at King's College Hospital in London which already houses some of the world's leading authorities on hormone replacement therapy. Their research has produced safe, easy treatments which help women in many countries. However, although the treatment has been thoroughly tested many GPs remain sceptical. They believe that the old wives' tales which cluster round the contraceptive pill also apply to HRT. Let's get this straight: *the contraceptive pill adds extra hormones to a woman's natural supply. HRT replaces missing hormones to restore you to normality*.

We have to bridge this gulf of ignorance and reassure GPs that HRT is safe and the benefits immense. I know from my own experience that it can do more to improve the quality of your life, your appearance, your energy and your happiness than pots of expensive face cream, a holiday in Spain or a complete new wardrobe of clothes. I could not possibly maintain my incredibly busy schedule without it. I wake up bright as a button every morning at 7 a.m., even though I rarely get to bed before 1 a.m. Each new year is a bonus and a challenge. I would like to share the benefits of HRT with as many women as possible. Indeed this book tells the story of hormone replacement through the experiences of the thousands of women we have already helped. It is a story which can transform your middle and later years and give you a wonderful new zest for life.

Teresa Gorman MP
February 1989

The Amarant Trust

Amarant: a mythical never-fading flower; a symbol of immortality and enduring beauty to the Greeks.

So WHAT IS THE AMARANT TRUST? In a nutshell, it is a charity which has been set up to promote a better understanding of the menopause, to support and expand research in this field and to make information and treatment available to many more women.

Its first project is to raise funds for a centre for mature women at King's College Hospital in London so that its pioneering work in this area can continue and progress.

We also want everyone to understand the biological changes which occur in women from their mid-forties; changes which can have a profound effect on their lives and which are a result of a natural decline in female hormones. Until recently they have been little understood – much less talked about. Even today many women suffer in silence through a distressing experience which saps their vitality and adversely affects personal relationships.

Advances in the techniques of hormone replacement therapy have produced remarkably beneficial results to which those few women who have been fortunate enough to have received treatment can testify. Research now reveals that HRT can also help to protect against many of the diseases of old age, and when combined with regular screening this can greatly enhance the prospects for women in their later years.

Ideally, the treatment should begin during a woman's middle years, but a woman is never too old to seek advice. It is a sad fact, however, that although the vast majority of women would benefit from this therapy, only six per cent actually receive it. Women and doctors need to be made more aware of the importance of such highly effective preventative treatment.

The Amarant Trust aims to make information about the progress made in this and related fields of medicine available not only to all women, but also to the general medical profession, who, in many cases, admit to wanting to know more but do not know where to turn for up-to-date advice about new techniques and prescribing procedures. It also plans to set up specialist centres where women can come for information and practical help.

Older women now comprise a fifth of the total population of Great Britain and this increases every year as we are all living longer. It is therefore more important than ever that we give them an opportunity to improve their quality of life. Mature women now play a greater part than ever before in society. Their contribution will be greatly enhanced, their health protected and their happiness ensured by the work of the Amarant Trust.

THE KING'S APPEAL

King's College Hospital is pre-eminent internationally in research into the menopause and its long-term effects. The Amarant Trust is appealing for £2 million to build and equip a new centre – the first of its kind anywhere in the world – where this unique and vitally important work can continue. A team, under the direction of Professor Stuart Campbell and Dr Malcolm Whitehead, has pioneered research into:

- Developing safer forms of HRT to replace the natural hormones lost through ovarian failure as women get older
- The use of ultrasound to detect early cancers
- How hormone loss affects sytems in the body especially bone metabolism

Over the last twelve years the King's unit has treated thousands of women and conducted trials to develop safe but effective methods of HRT. They have collaborated with the Institute of Obstetrics and Gynaecology, the Royal Post-graduate Medical School, the Imperial Cancer Research Fund Laboratories and the Cancer Research Campaign.

Current research is aimed at determining how hormone deficiency affects a woman's circulation, brain function and ageing in joints as well as influencing the health of skin, hair and nails. Also at determining the frequency of ultrasound scanning required for early ovarian cancer detection, and the possible use of ultrasound in the early detection of breast cancer.

Information about the work at King's is in demand all over

the world but the unit urgently needs facilities for research, teaching, clinical trials and treating patients. This would provide, for the first time in any country, a completely comprehensive service in one medical centre.

HRT is preventative medicine at its best and your support for the Amarant Trust will ensure a new era in health care for mature women.

1
Why the menopause doesn't have to be misery

THE BLACK FEELING of despair women often experience when they hit fifty or thereabouts is understandable. Suddenly life feels over, and they look back, wondering what have they to show for it. Isn't it downhill all the way from now on? They look in the mirror at hair that isn't glossy any more, skin that isn't plump any longer, a figure that may have thickened unbecomingly or thinned to scragginess, and compare themselves with either their own blooming daughters or young women they see in the street, and the gloom deepens. There's no cure or preventative treatment for age, is there?

Well, of course it is true that clocks can't be turned back; we are all going to get old unless we are struck down by disease or accident before our prime, but the gloom and despair aren't an essential part of ageing. They're neither necessary nor productive and simply spoil the rest of life which, believe it or not, can be just as interesting and fulfilling as when you were young. In fact, probably better because older women know themselves better, they are not so mortified at making mistakes, they're better informed and experienced, and quite often they have more money and more leisure.

This is the time for a second wind and to achieve personal goals instead of being at the constant beck and call of family. Edna Healey wrote her first book at the age of sixty and is in constant demand to talk to women's groups and appear on radio and television programmes; Mary Wesley started to write fiction at seventy; a company director learned to fly at fifty-eight; and a retired teacher is currently reading for her MA at sixty-nine. Everywhere you look there are encouraging examples of women who are determined to achieve their private ambitions. Don't write yourself off simply because you may have reached a significant birthday. Perhaps when life expectancy was so short that the end of life did indeed coincide with the menopause there was some justification for giving up. But today there can be twenty or thirty extra years of active life to look forward to. Imagine – you could take up a new career, become a painter, learn to sing or play the piano, enrol for an Open University course, study something esoteric that you have never had the time for before. Now it is your turn to indulge in a little selfishness and pursue your own interests.

But you won't want to plunge into all the inviting options if you are feeling dull and old, your energy is low, your bones ache, you no longer enjoy the loved feeling that comes from good sex with your husband, and you look in the mirror and see dry, brittle hair, and skin beginning to look like crumpled tissue paper. When you're in the grip of depression and despondency it is difficult to take a cheerful view of the future, but both can be banished. Just remember, it's *not your fault*. Your body is going through an upheaval and the chemistry is upset. Few of us take kindly to change. Moving house when you can't remember which packing case holds the essential kettle is a nightmare. Your body is 'relocating' some of its internal mechanisms and is having trouble getting its act together and meanwhile the usual smooth synchronization of its complex parts is temporarily out of order.

In middle age a very real physical upheaval is taking place akin to puberty. But just as it is fairly routine for many doctors to dismiss the pain and discomfort of periods as 'something you'll grow out of. Take an aspirin and go to bed with a hot water-bottle – you'll be all right once you start having babies', so too is the menopause, or 'change of life', regarded as something you put up with until 'all passion's spent' and you can subside gratefully into your rocking chair. One doctor practising in this country dismissed his poor patient battling with severe menopausal symptoms with the comfortless words, 'When they get to your age, women are *supposed* to rot.'

Like puberty and pregnancy, the 'change' is surrounded by myth and superstition, probably because originally doctors were invariably male, and women took their female problems to their more sympathetic older women friends who would respond with wise old saws – some of which, of course, worked. Even today doctors are overwhelmingly male, so it is small wonder 'feminine complaints', as they are sometimes contemptuously called, get short shrift.

Once the Amarant Trust was set up, and attracted a certain amount of publicity, the office was deluged by mail from women who suddenly saw a chance of getting some up-to-date, accurate information to help them with the bewilderment and depression they experienced at the onset of the physical change in their bodies, with no one censuring them for vanity. Here was somewhere where the menopause was not treated as a cruel music-hall joke.

The same agonizings cropped up again and again, and were repeated at the Amarant Trust's first conference in November 1988, when the Central Hall, Westminster was packed with over 1,500 women, all of whom sought advice about how to enjoy their middle years. One of the interesting things about this conference was that as well as the women who wanted to get at the facts about the menopause, along came women who had had hormone replacement therapy themselves. They were not seeking information and help. They came because the difference between the way they felt before treatment and after was so great that they had turned into evangelists. Billy Graham had nothing on these women; many of them had never stood up in public before, but all of them were motivated by their anxiety to share their experience with other women who were being discouraged, fobbed off with tranquillizers or told to pull themselves together.

Since, to judge from the Amarant Trust's postbag, not even the Albert Hall could hold all the women throughout Britain who want to know more, it seemed a good idea to pack into a book the questions most often asked and answer them as clearly and fully as possible without getting too mystifyingly technical. There's virtually a library full of papers setting out the research that has gone into menopausal symptoms and the virtues of hormone replacement therapy, and if you have the time and a dictionary to decipher the terminology you can research it all for yourself. But life's too short for most of us; we want to feel well and get on with our own work and preoccupations.

We owe it to ourselves to be clued up about our health.

Most women care about diet and nutrition, they have their hair looked after at hairdressers, and consult sales assistants on beauty counters in large stores about the best products for their skin and suitable make-up, but when it comes to their own health it is often a long way down the list of priorities. For some reason the menopause is still talked about in hushed tones, almost as if it were something shameful; women who would have boasted in their teens about the start of menstruation as a sign they were grown up dislike admitting they are menopausal. They fear it is official confirmation that they are old, ripe for a bus pass and a pension.

Hormone replacement therapy isn't a form of magic that will turn you into a young woman again. But in most cases it *will* improve the quality of your life and it *will* protect you against that disabling disease of old age, osteoporosis. It is preventative medicine at its best and before long, with luck, it will be prescribed as routinely as milk and orange juice are urged for babies.

The letter below perhaps best sums up how many women feel at this time – baffled, misunderstood by others and experiencing a panicky feeling that they are losing their grip:

'I'm forty-seven, and for the past two years my periods have been heavy and erratic. I feel my life is over. I'm no longer interested in sex, I am constantly tired, and weepily depressed for no reason. My doctor didn't seem very interested in my symptoms, muttered about "my age" and gave me a prescription for Librium. But surely today, forty-seven isn't old? And surely just dampening down, or suppressing feelings, which is what Librium seems to do, is not a cure but a palliative?'

No, forty-seven isn't old, nor is fifty-seven or sixty-seven or whatever age you like to mention, if you are reasonably active and mentally alert. This lady is clearly suffering from fairly common complaints. However, many GPs are either unable or unwilling to keep abreast of new developments in health and medicine.

One woman, for instance, wrote to the Amarant Trust saying:

*'I am sorry to tell you a long story but I have no one to turn to . . .
I noticed my hair and nails were dry and broken, sex was painful
for me, and my face was often red and flushed. I thought HRT
might help me but my doctor said, "Certainly not. It is a very
dangerous thing to do. You are just trying to turn the clock
back."'*

And another began a long letter saying:

*'At the commencement of the menopause I was treated for
depression. However, after completing my second course of
anti-depressants I began questioning this diagnosis. My experiences were pretty horrendous. I was totally unprepared for what I
experienced and, on reflection, rather saddened that I was treated
for so long for nerves.'*

Another woman was severely scolded, like a small child, by her GP who told her that requests for HRT, about which she had read so much in the press, were 'frivolous and dangerous. You cannot stay young for ever.' The Amarant Trust has had hundreds of letters like that, and whilst doctors are doubtless busy and overworked, the onset of the menopause causes as much mental misery and physical distress as some of the more familiar complaints listed in a medical dictionary, and should be treated seriously and sympathetically.

Put simply, the menopause is the end of menstruation, and a woman's childbearing years. Some women are confused by the word 'climacteric' which seems sometimes to be a replacement word. The climacteric is the winding-down process before your periods actually cease, the time between the possibility of pregnancy and the post-menopausal state when conception is no longer possible. It's a long, slow, natural process which usually takes two to five years. In the last few months before the final period a woman is 'peri-menopausal'.

In this technologically minded age, it might help to think of the body as a computer, being programmed at various stages of its life with software – the set of instructions that trigger various physiological changes. At puberty, for instance, the software programme is written so that a child gradually changes into an adult. This then makes it possible to produce babies. As we know, there's a stockpile of eggs in the woman's body, ready to be fertilized by the male sperm. The 'programme' has told the brain that the factory will have regular supplies of the hormone *oestrogen*, and another hormone, *progesterone*, will move in regularly to expel the unused endometrium (the womb lining) – or internal 'nest' prepared for the egg – if fertilization hasn't taken place, which is the process we know as a monthly period. The whole cycle repeats itself month after month in most cases, until the supply of eggs is used up, usually any time between the mid-forties and mid-fifties. Some women have more

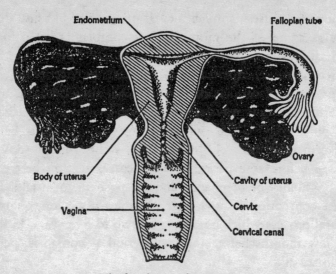

The female reproductive organs

eggs than others, just as some fruit trees are more prolific than others, so in their case the menopause comes later. Once periods have stopped for twelve months or more you can take it that you have completed the female cycle from puberty to menopause.

During the winding-down period, the menstrual flow can be very erratic. Sometimes scanty, sometimes so heavy that embarrassing flooding can occur almost without warning. The cycle can also lose its regularity. That is over-simplified of course, and probably repeating something you know already, but it doesn't hurt to have a brief recap from time to time, just to get the picture clear.

Of course, when the production of eggs is slowing, and the reproductive parts of the body are being prepared for redundancy, a new programme has to be written to give the

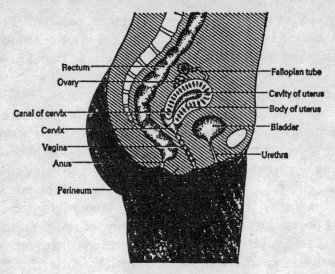

The female pelvic organs

brain a different set of instructions. Unfortunately, like the beginning of many computer programmes, there are often a few muddles and mix-ups. Until the 'bugs' in the system have been eliminated, and the new programme is running smoothly, the body's factory sometimes produces a lot of unwanted side effects including hot flushes, tiredness and depression. Quite often these symptoms are regarded by doctors as being all in the mind, and not linked to the menopause, which is why there is often an over-prescribing of tranquillizers. These can help in the short term to overcome anxiety and stress, but they are not long-term cures and do not seem to have any effect upon the daytime 'flushings' and the nighttime sweats.

Sooner or later, of course, the system accepts the redundancy programme, and we slide gradually into old age. But today, old age can go on for a very long time, because we are fitter, we eat more sensibly, we know the value of regular exercise, and many illnesses which at one time would have been killers have been disarmed or eliminated. Who wants to look or feel old when the whole depressing process of thinning hair, wrinkled, papery skin, stooped, rounded backs and restricted movements can be safely postponed for many years? We're not talking about putting back the clock, but of slowing down its relentless tick, which is why so many GPs dismiss efforts to do so as mere conceit. You can be pretty sure that if they started copious and involuntary sweating, forgot things, had a humiliating withering of sexual organs so that lovemaking was painful if not impossible, found themselves irrationally upset and irritable, their attitude might change.

When we can transplant hearts, replace kidneys and virtually wipe out tuberculosis, it's not surprising that medical science has found a way to alleviate or prevent the distressing symptoms of the menopause. Indeed, they've been working on the subject for many years, researching, testing and refining, until most doctors who have bothered to inform themselves of the background are pretty convinced that Hormone Replacement Therapy, or HRT for short, is not only highly effective but *safe*.

It has not been an overnight success story, but a slow, careful, painstaking build-up of collective knowledge which has produced the confidence to make pronouncements about safety and efficacy. Exhaustive double-blind tests on large groups of women in several countries have confirmed earlier results. It makes sense that if we can have spectacles to combat failing eyesight, all sorts of amazing orthodontic procedures to save teeth and smiles and continue efficient mastication, it is not outlandish to banish or alleviate disabling menopausal symptoms with HRT.

What HRT does is replace artifically the oestrogen we are no longer making naturally, combining it for part of the cycle with a second hormone progesterone. Like anything else, it must be prescribed properly and taken correctly because it's not like swallowing Smarties. And there were earlier scares about oestrogen *causing* womb cancer. Such scares have been nailed since it was found that what was missing from the therapy was progesterone. Once oestrogen and progesterone were combined they made a pretty formidable team and it has been suggested that between them they may actually *protect* women from womb cancer.

Perhaps the most important effect is the protection the therapy gives from osteoporosis, of which much more later (*see* Chapter 9). In addition, a happy extra bonus has been discovered in that women taking HRT have fewer heart attacks, and less arterial disease, and the most recent evidence is that HRT may help skin and hair health. Almost all the women who came to the Amarant Trust's November conference who had been using HRT for some time boasted that their breasts seemed more youthful, their complexions softer and their hair more glossy. No doubt it is because women dwelt, not unnaturally, on what they felt was an improvement in their looks that some doctors sourly dismissed HRT as merely cosmetic and, therefore, the women who sought it as vain.

Whilst HRT is undoubtedly beneficial to many women, it is a drug, and mustn't be treated with anything but respect. Just as some doctors *won't* give it to you, others prescribe it a bit too casually and sometimes do not check that the dosage and type is suitable for *you*. When it comes down to it, you must protect yourself by informing yourself so that you can evaluate how conscientiously you are being treated. Obviously a busy doctor is not going to take kindly to hectoring by a woman who may have read one loosely checked article in the popular press, so when suggesting you might be a suitable case for treatment, be tactful. If, as some of the Amarant Trust's correspondents have reported, your doctor dismisses it all as a mere youth drug, smile graciously and say he may be right but you would still like to be referred to a menopause clinic or a gynaecologist who has experience of HRT. No reasonable GP would refuse such a request.

It is important to have a thorough medical check-up before starting HRT and various tests should be done. Responsible doctors like to do an internal examination of the pelvic area, take a cervical smear, examine the breasts and record your blood pressure. Many family doctors are very happy to prescribe HRT; some are not – especially if you have had a medical condition which means that HRT should be given only by a specialist. In this situation, your GP may send you to an HRT clinic (if there is one in your area – there's a list at the back of this book) or to a gynaecologist, but if he is indifferent or actively hostile, your best plan, if you don't want to change your doctor, is to write to the Amarant Trust at 80 Lambeth Road, London SE1 7PW. (See also the list of telephone numbers at the back of the book.) But don't put up with misery; it's simply not necessary today. Whose life is it anyway?

2
What is HRT and how is it taken?

As we will say over and over again in this book – because it cannot be stressed to much – every woman is different and therefore her treatment must be individually prescribed. But don't put off consulting a doctor because you feel that since the menopause is a natural phenonomen you must grin and bear it. So is failing eyesight or hearing but you don't put up with that.

Sometimes, without trying to be alarmist, what you may consider as part and parcel of the menopause may be symptoms of a more serious disease. The menopause is so hedged about by myth and old wives' tales that a straightforward description of what it is all about is sometimes quite hard to come by. At this time of life, when periods are irregular and sometimes heavy, it is easy to dismiss unusual bleeding at an unexpected time of the month as 'the menopause'. Unexpected bleeding at the beginning, in the middle or at the end of your usual cycle must always be reported to your doctor, particularly if it is accompanied by any pain or occurs after intercourse.

If your local GP thinks that your description of how you are feeling squares up with the beginning of the menopause, he may be one of those doctors who are familiar with HRT and happy to prescribe it. It is available on the NHS so there should be no problem. If he's not too sure of all the latest developments, he may send you to a gynaecologist who has experience and understanding of HRT, or to a menopause clinic or Well Woman centre.

It would be a very good idea if we all kept a health log book. Doctors' records are not available to patients, and also many of us move about so much or change doctors so frequently that our records are not always clear or entirely comprehensive. Many mothers keep records of their infants' weight and immunization programmes, but as a rule we stop when the children are handed over to school. If we recorded our own illnesses, the dates, the treatment and drugs prescribed, any allergies to drugs experienced, pregnancies and any abnormalities, we'd make much better, more co-operative patients. As it is, when we get to a clinic or specialist we have to rely on shaky memory, when it is important to them to have an accurate medical history. A woman who has had a hysterectomy at a young age, for instance, may not have had her ovaries removed, which means she is likely to go on producing oestrogen. If she had had a hysterectomy, however, which included the removal of ovaries, she would have had a sudden, premature menopause soon after the operation, and oestrogen would be necessary, not only to alleviate any menopausal symptoms, but to avoid osteoporosis and certain arterial diseases such as heart attacks. Women who have an artificial or very early menopause are more at risk from osteoporosis and arterial diseases than those women who have a menopause in their fifties (*see* Chapter 8). Similarly, women with histories of gallstones, diabetes, high blood pressure or enlarged varicose veins may be prescribed different doses administered in different ways. If you can, arm yourself with notes of your various illnesses before you reach the clinic, together with the family medical history, because, as you know, there is a predisposition to certain medical conditions in families.

Before any hormone therapy is prescribed you will usually undergo some checks. Blood pressure and weight will be recorded, and you should have a pelvic and breast examination, plus the doctor will make a note of your family medical history. If the doctor thinks there are any reasons for special checks he may advise a mammogram and sometimes, though only rarely, a blood and urine test. Not until a complete picture of your health and background is collected can an effective programme be prescribed.

The therapy can be taken in a number of ways, each of which has its advantages and drawbacks. Again, your own medical history will do much to determine the method by which your therapy is administered, and your own wishes should be taken into account. Some women dislike the idea of a skin patch and prefer a pill; others find pill-swallowing difficult but would tolerate the patch; others are forgetful and need a regimen, such as an implant, that leaves little opportunity for missing a day. If you do miss a pill, or forget to apply a new patch, it is not the end of the world. Continue with the cycle as soon as you realize your mistake, but remember that forgotten pills or patches can cause irregular bleeding.

If you miss over a longer period, for instance if you go on holiday without packing your pills, you may find you experience a return of menopausal symptoms, and probably some bleeding or spotting. No long-term harm is done, but you must return to the correct time in the cycle, destroying the pills you forgot and not trying to resume them where you left off. Every month, the counsel of perfection is to 'oppose' oestrogen with progesterone, to avoid the thickening of the lining of the womb. If you miss the added progesterone days, it is not the end of the world – but don't make a habit of it.

THE DIFFERENT THERAPIES

Put simply, hormones are chemical messengers which deliver instructions to different parts of the body to perform an enormous variety of functions. If you think about it, overdosing on one particular hormone is likely to cause a disruption – that particular little chemical messenger is going to act like a bully, throwing its extra weight around and preventing the other equally valuable messengers performing their function properly. Therefore you want only the smallest amount necessary to nip in the bud the unpleasant symptoms of the menopause.

All hormone replacement therapies are only available on prescription. Your doctor can prescribe for you. However, some GPs may prefer to send you to a gynaecologist or a menopause clinic who may have more advanced knowledge than the average general medical practice, and the gynaecologist or clinic will suggest a dose and method for you. After that your GP may be prepared to give you repeat prescriptions, watch your blood pressure and carry out routine breast and internal checks.

What you must never do is accept a pack of HRT pills or transdermal patches from a friend. Dosage varies, and the therapy she is having may be quite different from the one you need.

When you first take HRT keep a note of your reactions. How soon did you start to feel better? Did any bleeding or spotting take place? Did you have a 'period'? Was it light, heavy, how long did it last? Did you feel nauseated? Did you notice a reduction in the vasomotor symptoms, i.e. the hot flushes and night sweats? These are all questions your doctor will ask you when you go back for your check-up, and it will enable him or her to judge whether the method and dose you are taking are right for you.

Here is a run-down of the different methods of hormone replacement therapy currently in use:

By mouth

Usually this takes the form of a pill a day, which towards the end of the monthly cycle is doubled with another containing progesterone. This second hormone, as we have said before, does the clearing-out job on the endometrium or lining of the womb. If the lining thickens regularly it encourages hyperplasia (an increase in cells), which in turn can encourage the growth of a cancer. Many years ago, oestrogen was given by itself for three weeks, with a fourth week free of any hormone because it was believed that the thickening would recede in the treatment-free week. This is now known to be incorrect and research has shown that by adding pro-gesterone a cleaner, more efficient job of shedding the thickened lining takes place. You do not need progesterone if you have had a hysterectomy.

The lowest dose of the oral oestrogen Premarin considered appropriate to alleviate menopausal symptoms and as a protection against osteoporosis is usually 0.625mg daily: Premarin plus progesterone is called Prempak-C. The lowest dose of Progynova needed to conserve bone is 2mg daily: Progynova plus progesterone is called Cyclo-Progynova.

When the progesterone pills have been finished, there is for the majority of women a 'bleed' like a monthly period. Sometimes this may be a little heavy when you start the therapy, but it usually settles down within a month or two. Unlike normal menstruation this is not an indication you are fertile again and could therefore become pregnant. Once you have reached the menopause you have passed your reproductive years. As mentioned elsewhere, between eleven to twelve per cent of women do not bleed; it isn't a danger signal, merely one that says the womb lining hasn't thickened to any appreciable extent. If you do not bleed, you must still take the progesterone.

Some women, particularly those who suffered from dysmenorrhea (painful periods) are put off hormone therapy by the idea of the monthly bleed, fearing that they will suffer pain and discomfort again, but this rarely happens. Bleeding is usually light, invariably trouble free, and easily coped with by regular tampons in four to five days.

Below is a list of the most usually prescribed preparations.

CYCLO-PROGYNOVA
Made by Schering, this utilizes human oestrogen (as opposed to synthetic, which is not generally used in HRT today) and

comes in a 21-day pack of tablets. You take eleven beige tablets containing lmg or 2mg oestradiol valerate, and follow them with ten brown tablets of oestradiol valerate 1mg or 2mg mixed with levonorgestrol 0.25mg (this is the progesterone). After this you have days twenty-two to twenty-eight when nothing is taken before starting the next pack. The disciplined woman who makes a diary note of when to resume the next cycle *and reads it* can cope with this method; the less organised or busily preoccupied woman could make a mess of the timing.

PREMPAK-C

Made by Wyeth-Ayerst this consists of a 28-day supply of numbered tablets in a blister pack. Every day from day one, a maroon tablet containing 0.625mg of oestrogen is taken. On day seventeen, this is partnered with a small pill containing norgestrel 0.15mg. 'Equine' oestrogens, which are extracted from the urine of pregnant mares, are considered to be longer-lasting. These packs are trouble free and leave little scope for mistakes through forgetfulness.

A higher dose, 1.25mg daily, is available for women with severe symptoms. This tablet is yellow.

TRISEQUENS

Made by Novo, this is a sequence of twenty-eight tablets packed in an attractive see-through plastic 'dial pack'. You turn the inner dial to the day of the week you commence the first tablet, a blue one containing oestradiol 2mg and oestriol 1mg, move on to the next day until the twelve blue tablets are used up. Then the dial delivers a ten-day sequence of white tablets containing oestradiol 2mg, oestriol 1mg and norethisterone acetate BP 1mg. The norethisterone is the progesterone. Finally, six red tablets are taken each containing oestradiol 1mg, and oestriol 0.5mg. It would be extremely difficult to make a mistake with this therapy, and it is of a convenient size to slip unobtrusively into a purse or pocket.

By implant

Another method of administering hormones is via an implant. This is a small pellet, usually containing six month's supply of hormones, which is inserted into the fatty layer of the tummy, thigh or buttock. It is inserted under a local anaesthetic and isn't painful unless you are one of those people who fear injections. The whole procedure takes under five minutes. The drawback of this system is that it is 'fixed' for six months, until the supply is used up. It means that changing the dose is impossible; if the dosage is too high for instance, it is difficult and complicated to locate the pellet and remove it, so the prescription has to be right first time.

Some GPs are happy to give implants but don't because it means an anaesthetic and an injection with a special instrument that delivers the implant. If this is the case, but he considers this method best for you he will probably send you to a clinic or a gynaecologist to have the pellet inserted.

Women who are forgetful and who can't make a routine of taking a pill every day prefer this method. So, too, do women who are made nauseous by the oral method. It also bypasses the liver, so it is used for women with gallstones or those with previous clotting problems. The implant technique can also be used to deliver two hormones, oestradiol and testosterone, which may help with menopause problems due to the loss of sex drive or sexual dysfunction.

As with other methods, however, twelve days' worth of progesterone in the form of pills is still necessary for women with wombs, so that women must remember to check their diaries.

A disadvantage of this method is that sometimes women experience a drop in their well-being as the oestrogen supply begins to diminish and they may harry their doctor or clinic for another pellet before the previous one is all used up. This can lead to a build-up of oestrogen.

By skin patch

A third method, which currently seems to be the most popular, is the skin patch – a little adhesive patch much like a see-through Elastoplast. At the time of writing it is also the newest, and research is going on all the time to develop further treatments.

This little patch contains a low, measured dose of oestrogen which is absorbed into the bloodstream directly through the skin, so again the liver doesn't have to cope with the hormones. It has to be replaced twice a week, and, as with other methods, progesterone tablets need to be taken for twelve days to make sure the endometrium is cleaned out each month. It is both simple and effective, and has the advantage of delivering lower oestrogen doses than pills or implants.

Drawbacks are few. Five per cent of women develop skin irritation and have to stop using the patch; absentminded women may forget to change their patch, and sometimes a hot bath or forceful shower may dislodge it. Otherwise it seems trouble free, and is probably the method which will be refined and developed most for the future.

Below is a list of the most usually prescribed preparations.

ESTRADERM

Made by Ciba–Geigy, this is the transdermal method of delivering hormones. In three strengths, of 25μg, 50μg and 100μg, the patches are packed in packs of eight. It does not include a progesterone, so this must be taken separately if the woman has not had a hysterectomy.

The adhesive patch, much like a translucent sticking plaster, is about the size of a 10p piece and contains a reservoir from which oestradiol is absorbed through the skin over a period of three and a half days. It has to be applied to a smooth, hairless part of the body, usually below the waist, where it is not likely to be rubbed by clothing. The best place is the buttock. It must *not* be applied to the breast. It should be changed as a regular routine, each time stuck to a slightly different area.

ESTRAPAK

By the same manufacturer as Estraderm, Ciba–Geigy, this is the same adhesive transdermal patch as above, but now marketed in a handy tabulated blister pack containing eight 50μg patches together with twelve 1mg norethisterone tablets.

The advantage of this product is that there is less likelihood of the user muddling up which day she should be taking which.

The transdermal patch method also means that the liver is

bypassed, and therefore lower doses of oestrogen are effective. It is one where most research is going on at the moment, and doctors are trying to find a way to include the progesterone in the patch to avoid separate, additional tablets. It is probable that a combined oestrogen/ progesterone patch will be developed and will become available in the UK.

Creams

There are also hormonal creams which can be applied locally, in measured doses of course (they come with a special applicator), to the vagina. They are often prescribed when sex is difficult because of lack of lubrication and atrophying of the vagina.

As we have mentioned before, once the brain receives the message that the body is no longer able to make babies, the reproductive equipment is discarded, left to degenerate, and the vaginal walls thin whilst the vagina itself shrinks and dries like a dry chamois wash leather. An oestrogen cream can regenerate the vagina, making it soft, supple and lubricated again. The cream is also absorbed into the bloodstream and therefore affects other parts of the body, although it isn't as effective as a skin patch or pills in alleviating hot flushes and night sweats, general depression and lack of energy. And because the cream contains only a very low dose of oestrogen there is no protection against osteoporosis.

The vaginal cream is the preferred route if no other menopausal symptoms are present and a woman is simply experiencing painful or difficult sexual intercourse. As a rule, it isn't a long-term treatment, and has to be watched because, as the dosage is self-administered, mistakes can be made. It is therefore important to be monitored *after* you have started on your therapy to make sure you are taking it properly and the dosage originally prescribed is doing its job adequately. It is also necessary to check to see that no adverse side-effects have developed. No conscientious doctor is going to give you a stronger dose than you need because hormones, though natural, are still drugs. Even though the oestrogen dose with the cream is low, it can still cause a build-up of the womb lining if used for many months. For this reason, some doctors add in progesterone tablets for twelve days every third or fourth month.

3
Is HRT *really* safe?

QUITE RIGHTLY, ever since the thalidomide tragedy, we've all been wary of drugs. Today's universal panacea may be tomorrow's sinister side-effect, and in an era when we are all concerned about E-additives to food, and growth-inducing hormones in cattle, shouldn't we be suspicious of any new treatment? Could it be possible that the doctors who say the unpleasant side-effects of the menopause must simply be suffered are not so much fuddy-duddy and unsympathetic as healthily sceptical?

'I've been a vegetarian since I was eleven, and have never taken things like headache pills. I grow my own fruit and vegetables organically and when rarely ill have usually resorted to herbal remedies from a naturopath.

'Unfortunately, nothing I've been prescribed by my naturopath has relieved the abnormal night sweats I have been having since the onslaught – and I use the word deliberately – of the menopause eight months ago. It is not unusual for me to change my nightclothes and bedding three times a night. I also have hot flushes and palpitations during the day, which are embarrassing as I am a sales assistant in a smart shop.

'I am so desperate that I am considering asking a conventional GP for HRT which my friend swears has saved her sanity, but I am not only terrified of interfering with the body's natural functions but also not at all sure this treatment is safe. In my belief, the menopause is a natural function, whereas administering hormones is not.'

No one would disagree with this correspondent that the menopause is a natural function. But lots of natural functions can cause problems. Think of babies teething, for instance. Nor would we be foolish enough to claim that hormone replacement therapy didn't have its opponents even today; there wouldn't be such a need for the Amarant Trust if everybody thought HRT a great idea. But the voices of opposition are muted in the face of overwhelming evidence that it is beneficial treatment, particularly for symptoms like those described above and as a preventative against osteoporosis. One could almost go as far as to say that it is only people who haven't kept up with recent developments on the subject who are against it.

In most hormone replacement therapies the oestrogens used are natural as opposed to synthetic, which is not the case with a great many other readily prescribed drugs. What we also tend to overlook today is that fifty years ago a woman's life expectancy was just over sixty years, so that suffering during the menopause was of a comparatively short duration. Now our life expectancy has stretched into the late seventies, and it is predicted that the next generation of women can expect to live until they are eighty-six. It seems ridiculous to put up with twenty or thirty years of old-fashioned 'old age' when it is no longer necessary. That doesn't mean we should try to hang on to eternal youth, but that we should avoid the thinning hair, dry papery skin and frequency of fractures that are so often associated with old age.

There was a scare in 1975 that HRT 'caused' cancer, but at that time oestrogen was used by itself, without the added progesterone. This caused the lining of the womb, the endometrium, to build up, resulting in a condition known as hyperplasia. Although not of itself cancerous, hyperplasia can lead to uterine cancer if neglected. The headlines flashed the story that women who took oestrogens were much more likely to develop uterine cancer, and not surprisingly confidence in HRT took a dive. What doctors had not realized then, fourteen years ago, was that progesterone was needed *as well* to induce the womb to shed the lining and so prevent the build up.

Today, only natural oestrogen is used for most HRT. It is usually prescribed continuously for the whole month, and then, during the last ten or twelve days of the cycle, progesterone is added. This has the effect of expelling the endometrium completely via a regular, light 'bleeding' like a normal period, although it doesn't mean that because you have a monthly bleed you are fertile once more. However, you don't have to have a bleed to be protected; approximately ten to fifteen per cent of women on oestrogen/progesterone will not bleed. This is normal and *safe*.

Because the birth-control pill contains oestrogen, hormone replacement therapy is often wrongly compared with it, and most women are aware of the scares associated with the Pill, like thrombosis for instance. But just as one air crash makes some people jump to the conclusion that air travel is dangerous, irrespective of the number of flights taking off every minute of the day all over the world without a problem, so the risks of the Pill have been exaggerated. In fact, for most women, having a baby is more dangerous than any side-effects of the Pill. In any case, the amount of oestrogen in HRT is much lower than that in the Pill, and is natural (although it is still produced in a laboratory) not synthetic, as in the Pill.

Recent research, on both sides of the Atlantic, has shown that properly prescribed HRT treatments not only alleviate menopausal symptoms but also prevent osteoporosis and appear to reduce heart attacks and strokes as well. But the key words are 'properly prescribed'. Each woman is different in her needs and it is important that the minimum dose necessary for obliterating the more debilitating symptoms of the menopause is prescribed.

Every woman who takes HRT should be followed up properly, either by her GP or at a clinic. This usually involves having the blood pressure and weight checked every six to nine months. Internal examinations should be performed every twelve to eighteen months, but cervical smears need not be taken more frequently just because HRT is being prescribed. For women over fifty years of age who have never had an abnormal smear, the recommended frequency of smears should be every three to five years. *Every* woman, however, whether or not she is taking HRT, should learn to examine her breasts every month. The doctor will also want to do this every twelve to eighteen months, but medical examination is no substitute for regular *self*-examination. Mammograms, a special type of breast X-ray, can detect early breast cancer and are increasingly being recommended to all middle-aged women over fifty years of age every three years.

Some people who abhor hormone medication may find that non-hormonal preparations may help alleviate flushing and sweating, but not usually in severe cases. These non-hormonal preparations include clonidine, Evening Primrose oil and Vitamin E. Whilst the preparations may help with mild flushes and sweats, there is no evidence that they alleviate vaginal dryness or help depression, anxiety, irritability, loss of self-confidence or prevent osteoporosis.

Certain diseases or a predisposition to a disease or condition can make hormone therapy more dangerous. Sometimes the extra risk is merely heightened, in which case you and your doctor must weigh up the severity of menopausal symptoms against the increased risk. So much depends on one's quality of life. If you are going through real torment, then you must decide whether the *possible* (not the probable) risks are worth taking in order to return to normal. No one, however enthusiastic they are about the benefits of oestrogen treatment, should attempt to influence a woman with real misgivings and a better knowledge of her own medical background.

WEIGHING UP THE PROS AND CONS

As we've said, there is hardly a therapy in the medical world that doesn't have its special cases, its exceptions and its disadvantages, and hormone replacement is no exception.

Cancer

We have already discussed the problems of oestrogen therapy, given by itself, and how it can cause build up of the womb lining (hyperplasia) in some women. Although not cancerous itself, hyperplasia can progress to cancer if neglected. Although the majority of the womb cancers caused by oestrogen are less invasive, and therefore are less dangerous, than those which develop naturally, no-one wants a treatment which causes cancer.

The addition of a progesterone to the oestrogen reduces the risk of womb cancer greatly. The protection given by progesterone depends not only upon the daily dose, but also the number of days it is taken for each month. Twelve days of progesterone is more protective than seven days.

Rightly, women are concerned about the effects of HRT on breast cancer risk. The incidence of breast cancer in women in this country has increased from one in seventeen to one in twelve during recent years. No one is sure why this has occurred: a part of the reason may be that women are living longer, and the risk of cancer is related to age – the older you are, the greater the risk. However there are lots of factors to be taken into account, like family history and dietary factors, for instance.

Because breast cancer is so common – and the majority occur in post-menopausal women, *every* woman should practise regular self-examination. Even then, some tiny breast cancers may not be felt and this is why mammograms (breast X-rays) are increasingly being recommended. Because HRT may accelerate the growth of a tiny breast cancer, mammograms are often advised before HRT is started. Five years of HRT does not appear to increase the risk of breast cancer. Much longer term treatment, fifteen to twenty years, has been reported to increase the risk slightly in some studies but not in others. This area is very controversial. Because the risk of spread to other parts of the body is reduced with early detection, mammograms are increasingly being recommended for *all* post-menopausal women, whether they are on HRT or not, every three years after age fifty.

With cancers of the ovary, the available data shows that oestrogen-only treatment does not increase the overall risk. There have, however, been three reports in the medical literature that oestrogen-only treatment may slightly increase the risk of one particular type of cancer, the *endometrioid ovarian cancer* (this has nothing to do with *endometrial cancer* which occurs inside the womb). These three studies have reported a small increase in endometrioid cancer with oestrogen-only treatment, but none of the observed increases achieved statistical significance, and the observations could be due to chance.

There is less documented research on oestrogen/progesterone therapy. There are no reports that the combined treatment increases this type of cancer. If anything, HRT would *decrease* the risk because it is well known that in younger women the contraceptive pill protects against ovarian cancer. Five years' use of the pill *halves* the risk of ovarian cancer for some years.

As far as cervical cancer is concerned, there is no hard evidence that either oestrogen-only or oestrogen/progesterone treatments change the risk of it occurring. Therefore, the frequency of cervical smears (every three to five years is recommended) is not altered if you take HRT.

Thrombosis

When the oral contraceptive, 'The Pill', was first introduced it contained a high quantity of synthetic oestrogen and an increased number of cases of thrombosis were reported. Thrombosis is due to clotting of the blood, and synthetic oestrogens seemed to cause the platelets of the blood to stick together, causing a clot or blockage in the arteries or veins, thus inhibiting the circulation. When a lane is closed on a motorway the remaining lanes become overloaded leading to long tailbacks, frustration, impatience and, often, accidents. The same thing may happen in your arteries and veins. If the platelets begin to clot, causing an obstruction, and if blood can't pass through freely, all sorts of problems are caused, the worst being a stroke or heart attack when the blood supply to the heart or brain is cut off, or a pulmonary embolus which cuts off the blood to the lungs.

Today's contraceptive pill has much lower doses of hormones, but these are still much, much more potent than the natural hormones in HRT. However, if you have a history of thrombo-emboli your doctor would probably be wary of prescribing HRT for you, particularly if you are damaging your arteries by being a heavy smoker. It depends very much on how serious your thrombotic disease was, whether it was associated with immobilization, how much you weigh, whether you smoke – and how fierce and miserable your menopausal symptoms are. The pros and cons have to be very carefully weighed. If you are feeling very wretched your doctor might start you on the very lowest dose possible and watch you like a hawk for adverse reactions.

But on the whole, the risk is slight. Women with small

varicose veins need not be prevented from taking HRT, but again, if the veins are very large and distended, their doctors would keep a special watching brief.

Hypertension, gallstones, hepatitis, diabetes

All these conditions may be exacerbated by HRT taken by mouth because the hormones would have to pass through the gut and the liver before reaching the circulation, irritating organs already damaged by disease.

There is a higher risk of **raised blood pressure** in women who are prone to this problem (those who are overweight, those who had high blood pressure when pregnant), but most doctors will be aware of this and if they prescribe oestrogen may suggest it is administered by the transdermal (skin) patch, or as an implant or cream. They will certainly want to keep a close watch on your blood pressure, and will tell women what warning signals to watch for.

Diabetics are not barred from taking HRT as long as adequate tests are taken before a course is prescribed, and the diabetes is well controlled. Whilst most conscientious doctors will make sure this is so, it is up to us to take responsibility for our own health too. Ask questions until you are satisfied with the answers. Don't be intimidated by a doctor's authority or afraid that the questions which worry you are too trivial for him. Once a diabetic embarks on a course of treatment, regular monitoring of blood sugar levels and urine samples should be a strict routine.

Oral oestrogens may also not be suitable for women who suffer from **gall bladder disease** such as gallstones, but here again, providing the treatment is not taken orally, and therefore doesn't have to pass through the liver, it may be safe. But, as before, careful checks are necessary first.

Smoking

It is well known that heavy smoking increases the risk of arterial diseases such as stroke and heart attack; oestrogen appears to considerably reduce the risk of such disease, and it can partially combat the effects of smoking. HRT has been found to reduce high blood-cholesterol levels, which are also linked to heart attacks. If you value your health and the quality of life, giving up smoking seems a small price to pay for the protection of your heart and lungs.

It is important to remember that current quantities of oestrogen in HRT are so small that they don't cause the upheaval they did a few years ago. Most research is devoted to seeing how far the dosage can be lowered in order to relieve the menopausal symptoms and give the undoubted protection against osteoporosis and arterial disease. When so many doctors 'in the know' are happy to prescribe HRT for their own families there doesn't seem to be a very substantial risk.

4

Can you have HRT treatment now, to prevent possible symptoms later?

THERE ARE QUITE A NUMBER of women who, having heard of HRT and its benefits, are anxious not to suffer as their mothers or older members of their family have done. They want to start the treatment now, whilst they are feeling all right, before depressing symptoms have a chance to creep up on them. This is a typical case:

> '*My older sister was prescribed HRT three years ago, more than a year after she had finished her periods. Until then she was in a terrible state – in fact, she was making such a hash of things that not only her job but also her marriage were in danger. I don't want to go through what she did, and now that I'm past fifty, I feel I should start similar treatment. At the moment my periods are as regular as ever, but they can't go on much longer, and I want to be prepared.*'

HRT, however, is not an immunization programme – it won't protect you from the effects of the menopause before you get there, as specific jabs will against diphtheria or cholera. It is a *replacement* of the hormone oestrogen once your body no longer makes it. If your periods are still normal and regular, you must still be producing both oestrogen and progesterone. If you weren't you wouldn't have a period. If your car's bowling happily along with the fuel gauge registering 'full' it would be pointless to call at a petrol station for a top up wouldn't it? You can't replace something you haven't lost.

As we have already said, the climacteric is the length of time it takes for the ovaries to shut up shop – in some women this time can last up to five years, although it is more usually two or three. Some women experience the occasional hot flush and night sweat *before* they are actually menopausal, i.e. before all ovarian activity has ceased. If pre-menopausal women are given HRT the bloodstream will carry too much oestrogen, both from the *natural* oestrogen provided by the still-functioning ovaries and the *added* oestrogen from HRT. This then produces fluid retention, breast tenderness, nipple sensitivity and leg cramps. Those are not symptoms you want to have.

In addition, whilst the body is at sixes and sevens coping with the gradual change-over from being fertile to ceasing egg production, the monthly period isn't always as regular as clockwork, whereas the administration of HRT is precise. This means the two sources of oestrogen/progesterone may not be synchronized and as a result breakthrough bleeding can occur.

Some specialists in HRT prefer not to give the treatment to their patients until the menstrual loss is very light and periods are becoming irregular. Of course, as we stress throughout this book, women's bodies vary, and in women who have very debilitating symptoms, an oestradial implant may be given which will suppress spontaneous ovarian activity. On the other hand, you may simply sail through the menopause without trouble, as an estimated twenty-five per cent of women do, in which case there would be no need to have HRT. Such women only notice they are menopausal when they suddenly realize they haven't had a period for some time. They have no hot flushes, no night sweats. It has just happened.

Oestrogen isn't necessary, as vitamins are, to your general health, but only if you are experiencing distress and discomfort similar to that suffered by our correspondent's sister. Women who don't have these problems, and particularly if they don't have a sexual partner (another menopausal symptom is a dry, tight vagina, but we will come to that) need not take HRT. It should be remembered, however, that oestrogen has been found to prevent the onset of osteoporosis, so before you decide it isn't for you, read Chapter 9.

HOW DO YOU KNOW WHEN TO ASK FOR TREATMENT?

There are women who experience symptoms such as hot flushes, irritability and headaches before their periods stop. Some experience periods that may occasionally be accompanied by pain and can fluctuate between scanty and flooding. This variation is often due to variable hormone production but any changes from the norm are worth watching; doctors would far rather you 'bothered' them with early symptoms than tough it out and perhaps store up future complications.

As a rule, once you experience heavy night sweats, day-time flushing, perhaps headaches and mood swings, you can take them as an indication that oestrogen production by the ovaries is beginning to fall and that the menopause is not far off. The best plan, throughout life of course, but especially approaching the menopause, is to put your health and fitness first. If you smoke, have another shot at giving up; watch your alcohol intake and keep it to the minimum and no more than a couple of glasses of wine a day; step up your exercise – you don't have to emulate Jane Fonda but half an hour's brisk walk a day is possible for most of us. Make a real effort to cut out biscuits, chocolate, cakes – a rule of thumb is avoid anything containing flour and sugar, which automatically means cutting down on fats, and is simpler to remember than obsessive diet plans. Try to aim for fifty per cent of your food intake to be fresh or raw – a box of thin sticks of carrot, celery, peppers, cucumber kept in a lidded plastic box in the fridge to divert you from cakes and biscuits when you are feeling 'snackish' is a good idea. If you keep up stocks of fruit and vegetables and don't even buy cakes, biscuits, crisps and all those convenience, ready-prepared meals which seem to have a creamy white sauce as a staple ingredient, you are well on the way to being in control of your weight. Postpone worries about what *may* happen to you during the meno-pause when, or if, you actually experience unpleasant symp-toms. That is the time when you and your doctor can discuss possible HRT.

5
HRT and the over-sixties

'I'm now eighty-eight and I could not be without my HRT. It makes all the difference to my feeling of well-being, my health and fitness. I also find, as do many of the women who write to me, that it helps to keep our skin soft and supple as well as making all the difference to our love lifes. The benefits are spectacular.'

Barbara Cartland

BARBARA CARTLAND SWEARS by it and has been taking it for almost forty years. Mae West took it up to her death aged eighty-five. Many women in their eighties who are active, attractive and still taking a full part in life may well be on HRT. That's not to say that all women of a certain age who retain their independence are on HRT, but there is a distinctly different quality about someone who has received this therapy and someone who has grown old naturally.

HRT is not a new-fangled treatment; in America, it is used by tens of thousands of women in their seventies and eighties who have taken it for twenty-five years or more. These women show a remarkably high level of general good health when compared with similar women who have not taken it.

Of course there are women in their seventies and eighties who are in fine fettle, but it is a sad fact that our nursing homes cater for large numbers of women who have become senile. These women have lost their ability to remember even the simplest things, such as how to light a gas stove, and as a result require full-time care. Is it worth living so long if that is to be our fate? In one small research study in America, senile elderly women were given HRT. The results were encouraging. They showed a marked improvement in their mental ability.

Lots of older women who read this book may say, 'I've been through the menopause and got over it. Should I think about taking HRT now that I'm in my sixties or seventies?' The answer depends on how likely you are to develop those scourges of old age – brittle bones (osteoporosis), strokes and heart attacks. These problems tend to run in families, so if your mother or close female relatives suffered from any of them you would be wise to talk to a specialist.

As a post-menopausal woman you have a much greater chance of fracturing your bones than a man of comparable age. And the risk rises steeply as the years go by. Additionally, the risk of arterial disease also increases after the menopause. The link between these problems and the loss of oestrogen is medically established. Furthermore, the risk is much greater than the risk of all kinds of female cancers. Over a third of all hospital beds are occupied by elderly women who are suffering from these menopause-related complaints. Think what the Health Service would save if we could prevent them.

If you have chronic pains in your joints HRT may well stop them. It's certainly worth a try. Women who know they are losing height because of fractures often complain of terrible pain in their spine. A curved spine will also eventually make breathing difficult because the lungs are constricted. Although HRT cannot put back the missing bone, it can halt the decline. That is why you should consider the therapy as soon as possible after the menopause. Remember, you are not taking a drug, but replacing something that nature has taken away.

Older women increasingly develop trouble in controlling their bladder. They also find it painful to spend a penny, and get a horrible stinging sensation and irritation as the skin in the area of the vagina dries out, splits and becomes infected. All these problems, however, respond well to HRT and creams are often applied locally for them.

Another demoralizing aspect of old age is losing your hair. HRT may improve the skin, hair and nails and certainly makes you look and feel better. However, HRT cannot reverse hair loss due to ageing as compared to lack of oestrogen.

One British doctor has said that HRT keeps you out of the hospital, the mad house and the divorce courts. Many women may say, why risk these problems if they can be prevented?

HRT will not make you live beyond your natural lifespan. But it can keep you in good health to the end. It is a preventative treatment at its best and you can do no harm in finding out whether it might be of help to you.

6

How long can you continue HRT?

EXPERIENCE OF prescribing hormones to deal with menopausal symptoms is not widespread, even now. But there are a significant number of women all over the world who have been having treatment for five years without ill effect, and providing you take an intelligent (as opposed to obsessive) interest in your own health, and are checked over by your doctor from time to time, the risks seem to be negligible.

'Short-term' treatment is considered to be anything from a few months to five years, and is started usually to combat the menopausal symptoms of night sweats, hot flushes, vaginal dryness, anxiety, irritability, loss of memory and concentration.

Some women are anxious not to continue treatment once their symptoms have improved in case there are any adverse effects in the future. Specialists at King's College Hospital Menopause Clinic reason that when the ovaries are in normal production the body makes its own oestrogen and progesterone naturally, without any ill effects, so why should it be different when the same hormones are prescribed once the ovaries have 'retired'? However, if you are one of those who dislikes the idea of taking medicines long-term you should remember that HRT can be stopped at any time, so long as you feel confident that you will not suffer again from unpleasant menopausal symptoms, and so long as you are not someone who is likely to develop osteoporosis. The choice is always yours. If you do stop, it will mean, of course, that the vagina will dry and degenerate again, but if you have no sexual partner or love-making is no longer of interest to either of you, perhaps this won't matter.

Like any other therapy, however, it is not a good idea to stop suddenly. You should taper off the treatment gradually, perhaps under the direction of your doctor. He may suggest you miss one day in three of oestrogen tablets, or don't replace the patch for the second half of the week. Then to miss two consecutive days or use three dermal patches in the month instead of four. Don't reduce the progesterone pills until you have stopped taking the oestrogen.

Whichever method you follow, you should monitor your reactions carefully, and check again with your doctor after a month or two to make sure everything is all right. Of course, if you have had an implant it will gradually be absorbed, but with implants you must continue the progesterone tablets every month until the periods finally stop: this can be as long as twelve months.

For such serious problems as osteoporosis, heart attacks or strokes, long-term treatment is probably essential. Unfortunately, for women who are already suffering from advanced osteoporosis or heart problems then HRT can't reverse any deterioration, although it may help slow its further progress.

Unfortunately no one knows yet the oldest age at which

HRT will be of benefit to prevent osteoporosis and these arterial diseases. Those women who start treatment before the age of sixty *will* be helped; those starting between sixty and sixty-five *may* be helped. For those who have already developed osteoporosis HRT is prescribed to stop further bone loss and the pain that goes with it. Women who start taking HRT later – sometimes in their seventies – do report an improvement generally. They feel brighter, sleep better and often their aches and pains improve, so it may be worth trying if you have these problems. One widow remarried at sixty-nine and found HRT caused her vagina to lubricate again and become soft and supple so that she was able to enjoy sex a second time around. A cheerful blow against ageism!

Another very good result from HRT is that it *can* prevent hardening of the arteries. Like osteoporosis this isn't a disease that can be reversed after it has happened, but it does seem that the major long-term benefit of HRT comes about as a result of the beneficial effects of oestrogens on blood vessels. It is only recently that such results have been documented and, as yet, this is not universally accepted by the entire medical profession.

It is recognized that women who take HRT for at least five years are protected against heart attacks and strokes, the number-one cause of death in women over fifty years of age. Research is also in progress to investigate possible links between senile dementia and other forms of psychiatric illnesses with oestrogen deficiency. Very preliminary studies conducted in the United States have suggested a small improvement with certain types of female dementia, in particular Alzheimer's disease. Anyone who has had experience of these two distressing illnesses would earnestly wish the link to be proven conclusively.

Preliminary results are also available for research studies which suggest that HRT may reduce the risk of rheumatoid arthritis – but at present it is early days and until such results can be unequivocally substantiated, HRT is not used as a treatment.

At the moment, the effects of oestrogen-only treatment on breast cancer are controversial. Some studies report that oestrogen-only therapy *increases* the risk of breast cancer, but others report a *reduction*, and yet others report *no change*; there is no agreement. If oestrogen therapy increases the risk, then it is important to know whether the increase in risk occurs with short- or long-term treatment or both.

A study from the National Cancer Institute in the USA has shown firstly that if the oestrogen-only therapy increases the risk, then this doesn't appear until it has been prescribed for five years. This study reported that extending the duration of treatment increases the risk still further, but the increases in risk reported by the National Cancer Institute did not – even at twenty years – achieve statistical significance. In other words, with oestrogen-only treatment there is *possibly* an increased risk.

This study also reported that the group of women who have a history *before* starting HRT of 'benign breast disease' (numerous breast cysts that aren't cancerous) are at greater risk, but then this same group is known to be at greater risk from breast cancer anyway.

There are, however, other studies in medical literature which have reported that five to ten years of oestrogen treatment does not increase the risk of breast cancer.

Additionally, whilst the National Cancer Institute study reported that women with previous breast lumps requiring surgery were most at risk, other studies have failed to confirm this.

When there is so much confusion between doctors, it is impossible for the general public to know what is going on. The conclusions that are valid are that breast cancer is common, whether you take HRT or not. It is related to age, and the older you are, the greater your chance of developing it. You cannot stop women developing breast cancer, but death can be prevented if it is detected at an early stage when cure is more likely. The best way to pick up early breast cancer is for every woman to examine her breasts each month to detect early signs. Mammograms are also recommended every three years in women aged over fifty. Whilst the government has recently stated its intention of establishing a national breast-screening programme, it may be some years before this is in full swing. Therefore, the availability of mammograms varies between different parts of the UK.

The effects of adding progesterone haven't been studied in detail to find out if, as with the lining of the womb, there is less risk. But as the breasts and womb respond in different ways, no assumptions can be made until carefully controlled studies have been made and evaluated. So far these have not been published. Therefore, based on current evidence, there is no need for women who have had a hysterectomy to take added progesterone.

Women who have to face surgery of any kind (even if unconnected with HRT – to have varicose veins removed, for instance) are sometimes advised to stop HRT six weeks before the operation because there may be an increased risk of blood-clotting with oestrogen immediately after the operation, and of course to ensure there is no clash with post-operative drugs the surgeon may prescribe. It may mean, of course, a return of the symptoms you were suffering from before the therapy, but once you have recovered from the operation, no doubt your doctor will give you the all clear to return to HRT.

7

You and your GP

ALWAYS REMEMBER that it's your body and your health and no one, not even your doctor, will have such a strongly vested interest in keeping it in good condition. That's why you must not allow yourself to be browbeaten if you think you need help. You are a client, not a beggar, so be prepared to stand up for yourself. The simple way to do this is to ask for a second opinion.

Doctors spend at least six or seven years on basic medical training, studying into the small hours to get their medical degree, and usually a number of years after that getting experience in hospitals and general practice before setting up on their own or joining a partnership. It is perhaps, therefore, understandable that they are not going to take kindly to a patient bursting into their surgery, waving a cutting from a popular newspaper or magazine (which may not have been thoroughly researched by the journalist involved) and demanding 'the treatment' described as a miracle cure. Particularly if 'the treatment' is for a non-fatal condition like the menopause. Doctors are also bombarded with numerous articles and papers in their own medical journals, as well as handouts from drug companies anxious that they should prescribe their products. It is small wonder then that the average busy and pressurized GP, who is perhaps upset by his inability to prevent a patient dying from some terminal disease, feels somewhat testy at being buttonholed by a grimly determined woman demanding HRT!

In an ideal world there would be enough money for the health service so that GPs could abandon their practices from time to time to take a refresher course in new techniques and therapies and to keep thoroughly up to date. But it is a far from ideal world and we have to rely on a doctor's own professional pride and interest to ensure he is abreast of new developments and treatments.

With something like the menopause, doctors quite rightly regard it as the natural phenonomen it is, like the onset of puberty. But too often they expect women suffering serious discomfort to stoically soldier on. Some women don't have any problems, they point out, so the ones who are making a fuss are probably self-centred hypochondriacs simply wanting a bit of attention. A recent letter to The Amarant Trust from a distressed woman read:

'I am suffering severely. I have erratic and profuse bleeding, so much so I flooded the floor of my supermarket to my intense embarrassment. My GP says this sort of situation is normal and I must accept it.

'The obvious step would be to change my GP but in this town it is virtually impossible. If you approach any of the other practices they tell you their books are full and that they do not accept transfers.

'My long-suffering husband came with me to my doctor when I went to him a third time, to reinforce my explanations of how

dreadful I felt but he merely suggested psychiatric counselling, a prescription for Librium and told me to pull myself together. "You are not the only one," he said.

'Finally, I got to see a gynaecologist after some months of badgering, and was relieved to find I was neither mad nor psychosomatic but suffering from a hormone imbalance because I was peri-menopausal. Unfortunately I still have to attend my GP for a renewal of the hormone prescription and each time I am treated to a stern lecture on the financial drain I am on the health service. The fact I feel like a normal human being once more cuts no ice.'

This poor lady was obviously particularly unlucky, but her doctor's prejudice is by no means as uncommon as we would wish. Another woman wrote to The Amarant Trust saying:

'I am at the moment taking HRT but it has been a long, hard battle to get it prescribed and I feel sure that once this course is finished my doctor will not prescribe any more.'

And a third wrote:

'My doctor will not give me HRT as he says it causes cancer, so I must go on with these debilitating hot flushes and feeling my life is at an end as I am too embarrassed to go out.'

Unfortunately the menopause, like mothers-in-law, has always had a bad press. There are the tasteless music hall jokes, the implication that if women in jobs are bad-tempered and irritable it is due either to their periods or lack of them. Yet bad-tempered men are treated with respect: 'He must have a lot on his mind', it is assumed. It is only in the last years that it has become generally accepted that the distressing side-effects of the peri-menopause (the time before you have your final period) and post-menopause (after your ovaries have stopped producing eggs and you have stopped your last period) have an actual chemical base. After thirty years of continuous research we now know that most unpleasant menopausal symptoms can be alleviated, but many doctors trained before research became widely known. This whole book is about putting you in the picture, so that you can be informed about your own health and well-being. We probably need another one for doctors – if they could find time to read it. But try to avoid having open warfare with your doctor. It isn't always easy to change your doctor in a small community as one of the correspondents above pointed out, so that it is better if, when seeking medical help, you do so with tact, and an understanding of his pressures. At the same time, you have a right to want to feel well, to believe that your years ahead can be active and interesting, so don't be afraid of combining your tact with firmness. Smile sweetly as you mention that you *know* there are therapies to improve the way you are feeling now. Explain you didn't want to bother him unduly, but you have now had an opportunity to read widely on the subject of menopausal symptoms. It is nothing to do with vanity and wanting to stay young for ever, but it is to do not only with the quality of your life but also the quality of the lives of your friends and family who can't help but be affected by your behaviour. At the moment, you might explain, you are simply not in control of either your physical or emotional states.

Fortunately, most doctors are reasonable and will concede that you may have more motivation to find out about what new therapies are available than he has. He would also have to agree that anyone would need to be blind, deaf or supremely indifferent not to catch health programmes on television or radio, or to read medical updates in some of the more serious women's magazines and newspapers. If your doctor sees that your manner is not aggressive, but that you are clued-up and that you are having such severe menopausal symptoms that it is difficult to carry on a normal life, he will no doubt prescribe for you or, if he is big enough to admit his own limitations of knowledge in this field, refer you to a specialist.

Great Britain is one of the few EEC countries where a referral letter from a doctor is usually necessary before you can see a specialist. Whether this will change in 1992 remains to be seen. Faced with a refusal from an implacable doctor, most British women would quail and give up, but in fact it is your right to ask for another opinion, although doctors sometimes choose to interpret the NHS rules as being up to *them* to decide whether a second diagnosis or opinion is necessary.

Women who can afford private treatment can often bypass an obstinate doctor by going direct to a gynaecologist recommended by a friend, but this has repercussions. The gynaecologist will usually want to write to your GP to tell him the result of the consultation, so cannot keep your visit a secret. Funnily enough, however, many GPs are just as much in awe of a specialist or consultant as most of us are, so that they will generally content themselves with an irritable mutter or two but continue with your prescriptions!

If your doctor is very old-fashioned and lacking in understanding that he scolds you for attempts to 'turn back the clock' and is openly hostile, then it may be time to seek another doctor. You can do this by writing to your local Family Practitioner Committee and asking for a list of NHS doctors. Alternatively, if for some reason changing your doctor is not practical, you might find the nearest Family Planning Clinic helpful. Like the Amarant Centre, they have someone who can prescribe and supervise treatment or, if not, they can give you a referral to a gynaecologist.

It was because of the problems women had in obtaining treatment that the Amarant Trust came into being. One of the principal aims of the charity is to encourage the setting up of more specialized clinics to make HRT treatment more widely available. Another is to raise money to train more doctors about the menopause, including up-to-date techniques of HRT.

The first Amarant Centre has been set up at the Churchill Clinic, 80 Lambeth Road, London SE1 7PW, and is supervised by specialists from King's College Hospital Menopause Clinic, which has more than fifteen years experience in this field and a world reputation for research into the problems of menopause.

There is a charge, because the Centre is non-profit-making, is registered as a charity and has no Government funding. Quite often, after the initial consultation, some GPs will repeat the hormone prescription on the NHS. However, they are under no obligation to do this.

Obviously not everyone can visit the Amarant Centre, that is why there is a list of Well Woman and Menopause Clinics at the back of this book. Those which are NHS funded are marked.

8

Why sex suffers at the menopause

RELATIONSHIPS quite often become severely strained during the menopause. A woman may feel she is losing her appeal, that she's old, and that it is undignified and incompatible with her mature status to feel any sex drive. Or she may become more susceptible to flattery and romantic words from a personable man who will supply the reassurance she needs about being still attractive, perhaps because her husband has settled into a dull routine and no longer seems to notice her. Men, too, start doubting their previous capacity to attract. They will frequently go out of their way to chat up younger women, to prove to themselves they are still appealing.

Psychologically, both partners are vulnerable to the lure of new friendships, but are really looking for confirmation that they are still interesting and attractive, and count as individuals. Physically, it is probably related to the lower levels of the male hormone, testosterone. This is another hormone, present in both sexes but particularly in men, which diminishes with age. Older women lose not only oestrogen but also testosterone, and with it often their sex drive. They're not so interested in physical sex themselves and become

70

impatient with their husbands who still are, thinking they should be 'over that sort of thing at their age'. The subsequent rebuffs are hurtful to a man already apprehensive about getting old.

When the psychological and the outward physical signs of ageing combine, both partners begin to lose self-confidence. Women in particular tend to have poor self-esteem and a low body image. To them every advertisement seems to centre on a lean, lithe, youthful body. How can a fifty-plus woman compete? We're constantly fed a diet of glamour and often forget that these models of perfection are only achieved with the aid of a battery of make-up artists, hairstylists and wardrobe masters, not to mention body-contouring experts and cosmetic surgeons. Is it surprising therefore that the ordinary middle-aged woman begins to feel inadequate and inferior?

A hormonal check-up and a course of treatment could prevent these and similar worries, but unfortunately many people consider such problems all too trivial, vain if you like, and can't bring themselves to discuss them with a doctor. And it has to be said that you have to be lucky to get your doctor to appreciate how much such concerns distress you.

It's sad but true that a great many divorces take place in the middle years of marriage and perhaps the waning of sexual pleasure and the fears of ageing have a lot to do with it. The early days of a partnership require adaptation and change, but the later years need freshness, stimulation and, above all, reassurance. After years of living together it is so easy to take each other for granted, to no longer be surprised.

It isn't a promise but it is a fact that at the menopause some women experience an orgasm for the first time. Perhaps the relief of no longer having to worry about pregnancy is one reason. Another may be that for the first time since early marriage they can be alone with their husbands. Children have grown up and left, there is no longer the pressure to climb a career ladder, and they have a little more of that precious commodity, time.

Unfortunately, the reverse side of the coin is that sex can become physically more difficult and painful. The vagina doesn't lubricate as easily, its walls become thin and more vulnerable to damage. The fear of pain and discomfort leads to further tension, and unless a husband is very understanding, the rift between a couple widens. Here is a letter from a woman has encountered just such a problem.

'At fifty-seven my sex life is absolutely nil whereas until seven or eight months ago it was highly satisfactory. I get desperately tired now, I have pains in my head and knees, and I seem to have a permanent chip on my shoulder. My husband has been kind, but his patience is wearing thin and he is as bewildered as I am. He simply tells me to take it easier – I do have quite a demanding job as well as a home to run – but I've managed both for years, without problems, why should I find things so difficult now?

'I think I would have gone soldiering on, hoping I would pull out of this "slough of despond" sooner or later if it weren't for the fact that I fear my husband will look for another woman. We have always enjoyed a very full sex life, and for both of us, but particularly for him, lovemaking was very important, but now it is virtually at an end and I know he feels bitter and frustrated. It's embarrassing even to write it down, and I certainly couldn't talk to my doctor about it, but the last few times that we tried to make love, quite a few weeks ago now, I was so dry that penetration *was difficult and I experienced actual pain, as if I were a virgin. I believe my husband thinks I don't want him and once or twice this has caused him to lose his erection, which made him angry and upset. I did try a particular jelly, it helped a bit but he still thinks the dryness is because I am no longer interested in him.*

What we sometimes forget in the preoccupations of every-day life, is that physical contact is important to us all. People lose the ability to discuss their feelings and forget that a warm, outward demonstration of affection – a spontaneous cuddle, a smile and a squeeze of the arm – can diminish fears and produce the right climate for an open discussion of what is wrong. Men aren't indifferent to women's moods but they are sometimes baffled by the mood swings produced by the chemical changes going on in our bodies. If we don't understand them properly, how can they?

Even if you are suffering from loss of libido, or feel just plain rotten, somehow you have to convey that your love is unchanged. The whole business of female chemistry is mysterious and bewildering to many men. They are embarrassed by it, perhaps because they haven't had adequate sex instruction, and at this time they need reassurance that your love and interest in them are as strong as ever, just as you need to take their goodwill and understanding for granted.

There's so much discussion about medical problems on television and in the press that we sometimes assume everybody knows all about everyday health problems, but they don't. Some people are too squeamish to want to know too much about illness and bodily functions, and others don't know where to go for information, particularly when there is no obvious, specific disease. The woman whose letter is reproduced above must explain to her husband that she's going through a bad patch physically, that she has been abnormally tired and depressed, and that it looks as if she needs medical help to get over it. She must assure him that she is going to take positive action to get better right now because she has not enjoyed these past few months any more than he has. Her next step is to stifle her embarrassment – after all, as she says herself, she believes her marriage to be at stake, so she has a strong incentive to overcome her qualms, and go to her doctor to tell him how she feels. Don't spare his blushes or yours. Today few doctors believe that emotional problems don't have a connection with one's physical condition, and taking her age and other symptoms into consideration, it seems highly likely that she is suffering the effects of the menopause. If it makes her feel any better she can ask her doctor to refer her to a woman doctor, but she must not delay. Help is available, all she has to do is ask for it.

What we don't always realize is that once a woman's production of oestrogen slows down, the vagina is no longer necessary and it starts to shrink, dry up and even to change shape. It's all part of the body's clever programming. It is no longer in the business of making babies, so the lubrication needed to encourage and ease penetration by the penis for fertilization of eggs is unnecessary. Nature seems to have overlooked the provision of lubrication for straightforward fun and enjoyment of sex for its own sake!

If you are only just into the menopause, and have had a regular and active sex life, the atrophying of the vagina is slow, and the dryness can be counteracted by KY-jelly or a similar lubricant. But usually, vaginal oestrogen cream, or the full HRT programme of oestrogen combined during part of the month with progesterone, will quickly restore the moisture and youthful flexibility of the vagina – and of course, the normal, or even enhanced, enjoyment of sex. This can happen even some years after the menopause, so never believe it is too late. If you still want a full sex life, then HRT in one form or another will help to eliminate problems. However, remember the cream still contains hormones which are absorbed into the bloodstream, so it must not be confused with the spermicidal jellies and creams sold chiefly to enhance lubrication.

There are also other sexual problems associated with the menopause. As we've said, some women experience a loss of libido (sex drive) during the menopause – real or imaginary. Lovemaking seems a drag and an unnecessary chore, obviously a hurtful attitude for partners. Others, to their surprise, find their libido is increased. On the other hand, age and familiarity may have caught up with one's partner and new enthusiasms have to be introduced to freshen the relationship. If you're experiencing new interest in sex, but it all seems one-sided, then you have to shock and surprise your partner into a new awareness of you as a still-attractive, desirable woman. We don't always realize men need encouragement and a sense of romance and excitement too.

Real loss of libido is frequently linked to the fact that sexual intercourse is more difficult, not only for the reasons mentioned above but because the vaginal walls have thinned during the decrease of oestrogen, and as a result they are much more liable to injury and irritation, called atrophic vaginitis. Vigorous thrusting by your partner can cause small tears, which become the sites for infection and inflammation. Vaginitis can thus be a problem for older women as it sometimes is for women in early marriage.

If you are experiencing a lack of interest in sex and wish to do something about it, you may find your gynaecologist recommends a hormone implant. This is a straightforward insertion of a small pellet, about the size of an apple pip, in the fatty layer of the abdomen, thigh or buttock which slowly releases oestrogens over a period of about six months. It is no more complicated than having an injection and, as the pellet can be combined with testosterone, the male hormone, libido often improves. Very rarely the testosterone may cause a slight increase of facial hair but this will disappear when the testosterone implant wears out.

Even with improved sex drive, efforts to renew a close, sexual relationship may be stultified by shyness. Taking more rest, giving priority to pleasurable things like listening to music or taking the trouble to plan a meal with wine and a candlelit table can help to set a romantic mood. Develop sensitivity not only to your own moods and what gives you pleasure, but to what seems to please your partner. Put your antennae into overdrive to pick up your partner's vibes.

Some women are all too relieved when they become menopausal as it gives them an excuse for giving up sex altogether. These are often the women who have always had hang-ups about sex and never particularly enjoyed it anyway. They like to use the excuse of reaching middle age to put away sex, rather like packing toys into the attic, but for these women it isn't the menopause which is at fault but their own inhibited attitudes. This is all very well if they are married to men who are similarly disinterested, who prefer golf or homing pigeons as pastimes, or those men who have long been disappointed and resigned to their wives' lack of sexual response and whose participation in the act was routine and uninspired. But if the men are still keen on sex these wives will probably be facing marital problems of one kind or another before very long.

Sometimes, when marriage has jogged gently along in a routine way, with job worries and children preoccupying both partners, it takes a little while to come to terms with the new changes going on. You are thrown on to your own resources of conversation and entertainment again; there are the new physical sensations to take aboard when both partners are undergoing a hormonal change, and it quite often happens that they are shy of each other, not quite sure of how to behave together any more. One woman wrote to us saying:

'I'm ashamed to say I really don't know much about my body at all. I had a hysterectomy some months ago and nobody has explained to me, in words I can understand, what is happening to me. My husband is terrified of hurting me, and I am very shy. As a result, sex is infrequent and not very satisfactory.'

It is depressing to learn this woman was not offered more information about her hysterectomy. Presumably, she had a post-operative check-up and everything had healed nicely, or further treatment would have been necessary, but it would have helped if she had asked the gynaecologist to discuss her sexual anxieties. It is always a good idea to know what is going on in your own body so that you can make informed decisions when you are offered alternative treatments, or ask intelligent questions if you feel there are too many blanks in your knowledge.

Don't think it is too late to learn all over again about sex. If you have problems, it could be a good idea to talk to a sex therapist – the organization called Relate (which used to be the Marriage Guidance Council) have trained sex therapists to whom you could be referred, and who can help you understand your body and your sexual reactions. They set aside an uninterrupted hour of time to let you talk and pour out your worries and inhibitions. They are not judgemental, are totally discreet, and draw on a great deal of experience and training. Relate is independent, non-denominational and entirely voluntary. If you value a warm, intimate relationship and you are having some temporary difficulties, it is worth seeking professional help. You will find your nearest branch listed in the telephone directory, but in case of difficulty, send a sae for a list of centres to Relate, Herbert Gray College, Little Church Street, Rugby, Warwickshire CV21 3AP. There are also some helpful books worth reading listed at the end of this book.

9
HRT and osteoporosis – the long-term benefits

THERE IS A big difference between osteoarthritis and osteoporosis though, obviously, as the names indicate, they both concern bone. Osteoarthritis, a form of arthritis in which the cartilages of the joint and adjacent bone are worn away, can attack after an injury, or from sheer wear and tear on the joints. Both men and women suffer from it, particularly men who have damaged themselves in sporting accidents. HRT does not have any beneficial effect upon this disease except in a very small number of cases where, at the time of the menopause, a woman suddenly develops joint pains in her fingers, wrists, elbows and perhaps shoulders. HRT relieves the pain for some of them, but doctors are not clear why this should be so.

Osteoporosis, on the other hand, is an insidious disease that creeps up on us over the years. Bones become porous because of a loss of bony tissue and slowly waste away, at about the rate of two to three per cent every year due to a process called resorption. Unfortunately this wastage gives no outward symptoms, until fractures start to occur. By that time, it may be too late to be put right. You can't actually put back bone which has been lost.

Osteoporosis will affect one man in twenty, though for women this figure rises to one in two. The risk is greater if there is a strong family history of the disease – for example if your mother or grandmother suffered from this condition. You may also be at risk if you had an early menopause or removal of the ovaries. Woman who are over forty, who drink more than five or six cups of tea or coffee a day, who rarely exercise, who are small-boned and pale-skinned, and who hated milk at school, are also more at risk, particularly if they also smoke or indulge heavily in alcohol. It should be remembered, however, that everybody suffers bone loss as they get older, the high-risk group merely gets it earlier and more severely than the rest of us.

Osteoporosis is a crippling disease. Next time you walk to the shops count how many elderly women you see with the tell-tale 'dowager's hump' – that unattractive outward curve at the nape of the neck – hobbing along supported by their shopping carts. Probably all of them are suffering from the creeping disability of crush fractures of the spine, a condition that is progressive if it isn't halted. After a while there is a tendency to break wrists and hips in a simple fall, which later cause chronic disability. Some women have such severe bone loss that they are bent almost double, which makes movement difficult and painful and leads to all kinds of breathing difficulties as the chest wall is compressed.

Statistics in the UK show that in 1985 over 35,000 women were admitted to hospital with hip fractures, 20,000 of whom died or who became permanent, dependent invalids. The visual evidence of creeping osteoporosis is all around us – women bent and deformed by disintegrating bones and frequent fractures. Once you are aware of it it sometimes

HELP THE WORK OF THE
AMARANT TRUST
BY BECOMING A MEMBER

Our information pack includes a list of Menopause clinics throughout the country, together with copies of our newsletter **Feeling Good** and our booklet **Change for the Better.** Send a cheque for £5.50 (inc. p&p) made out to the Amarant Trust.

The Amarant Trust is a charity and needs your financial support. Annual Membership (which includes the £5.50 information pack) costs £12. It keeps you up-to-date on research through our regular newsletter and entitles you to individual advice. We would also like to hear from you if you can help us with fund-raising or setting up a support group in your area.

Please tick the appropriate box(es) and return to the Amarant Trust, 16-24 Lonsdale Road, London NW6 6RD.

- [ ] I enclose £5.50 for an information pack

- [ ] I enclose £12 (minimum) membership fee

- [ ] I would like to help in fund-raising/starting a support group in my area.

- [ ] I enclose a donation of £ .... towards the work of the Trust.

PLEASE WRITE CLEARLY

Name ....

Title .... Age ....

Address ....

....

.... Post Code ....

Daytime Tel.No. ....

Date ....

Amount enclosed £ .... (please make cheque payable to 'The Amarant Trust').

seems as if every other woman over the age of sixty is a sufferer. It is not a disease to dismiss lightly, an inevitable price for living to old age, for women suffering from osteoporosis frequently become so disabled that they are unable to look after themselves and are condemned to life in an institution.

The tragedy is that with knowledge, there is a lot you can do to ward off the problems. One of the marvellous things about HRT is the effect it has on bone – which is perhaps of more value than its original role in relieving distressing menopausal symptoms. To a very small extent, it may actually restore some bone mass, but more importantly it prevents further deterioration. It's like shoring up an old, historic building with pinning and discreet RSJs to stop crumbling and erosion. As one of our letters from a 78-year-old woman said:

> *'The discovery that I was suffering from osteoporosis (of which I had never heard) was a great shock to me and came really too late for me to benefit from HRT as by then a bone scan showed I had lost sixty-eight per cent of bone density. But by taking hormone tablets every day the loss has been stabilized.'*

It has been conclusively proven that oestrogen prevents bone loss, a fact the following letter brings home:

> *'My mother is now in her eighties, small and frail and completely bedridden. When she was thirty-eight she had a hysterectomy (including removal of the ovaries) and it was about two years later that she started to have troubles. I came back from three years of living in Australia and was shocked at how stooped she was,*

and as a result not nearly as tall as I remembered her. Soon after she suffered her first major fracture. I'm not married, so I made my home with her, and ever since she has had one fracture after another – one merely through a coughing fit!

'*Now I know that bones need calcium and perhaps my mother didn't have enough when she was young. Obviously her early hysterectomy aggravated her condition, because isn't it true that oestrogen stops excessive absorption of bone. I am fifty-two and having mild menopausal symptoms, such as not-too-severe hot flushes, irregular and heavy periods, which don't bother me too much, but I am terrified of ending up like my mother, especially as I haven't a daughter to look after me.*

'*I've read about hormone replacement therapy but would it be suitable for me, even though I have not had children, or married, and can't say I am suffering much torment so far? It sounds faintly ridiculous to go to my doctor and say "Can I have some treatment even though there's nothing really wrong with me?" I don't want to bother him unnecessarily, besides he'll probably think I'm either mad or a hypochondriac.*'

Oh dear, it does seem tragic that we are so frightened of bothering doctors, even with very real fears, that we are prepared to suffer, or worry, in silence. Most doctors are normal, sympathetic creatures and though we may moan about a small minority who dismiss worries about the menopause by attributing them to vanity and as something a woman has to put up with, most would appreciate the common sense shown by this woman, especially if osteoporosis is in the family, since it can be hereditary.

In this case, it is likely that the mother's ovaries were removed at the time of her hysterectomy. Nowadays, some surgeons try to preserve the ovaries in young women, unless of course they are diseased too, because they will go on producing oestrogen which protects against bone loss, and there won't be the sudden bodily shock of an artificial menopause. Other surgeons remove the ovaries of women in their forties to prevent against later ovarian cancer: these surgeons then recommend HRT.

Women who have a surgically induced menopause or who have a particularly early one are deprived of oestrogen too soon and are left unprotected from oesteoporosis. Nowadays, of course, providing they seek treatment, they can be given oestrogen which will prevent the insidious advance of this bone disease.

The Amarant Trust receives many letters on this subject. Another correspondent wrote:

'Five years ago a bone scan revealed that I was suffering from osteoporosis. In addition, vaginal dryness made sexual intercourse impossible and my marriage was virtually on the rocks. (I am now divorced.)

'My GP gave me a prescription for calcium lactate tablets but told me HRT was frivolous and dangerous. "You cannot stay young for ever." I have since approached several other doctors but the answer is always negative. What can I do? I feel so helpless and depressed, especially when I think of my mother who suffered five fractures and died as a result of one.'

This Liverpool woman has tried to alert doctors to her menopausal condition but to no avail. If HRT treatment had been begun five years ago it could have helped considerably to halt the progress of her osteoporosis and might have saved her marriage. It is still possible to prevent further erosion of the bones if she starts on oestrogens now but she won't be able to replace the bone mass she has already lost to any great extent.

WHAT YOU CAN DO TO MINIMIZE THE RISK OF OSTEOPOROSIS

Slim, small-boned 'English Rose' complexioned women are more prone to osteoporosis than dark people, so, too, are those who have had a hysterectomy, which has left them without ovaries, and those women who stopped menstruating before their mid-forties. Smoking and heavy drinking, as do so many other diseases, adversely affect osteoporosis. A sustained and determined effort to stop smoking altogether and to at least cut down on alcohol intake therefore makes good sense. As a rough guide, heavy drinking amounts to three to four glasses of wine a day. It is thought, however, that the odd glass of wine helps metabolize food, so if you enjoy a drink it is unnecessary to cut it out completely.

It doesn't matter whether you have been married or not, or whether you've had children or not, even if you're female – because men can suffer from osteoporosis as well. In their case, they are usually much older than women before it becomes debilitating, and it doesn't seem to strike as frequently or as severely. Women have smaller frames than men, so that once they stop producing oestrogen naturally, their bone loss quickens, and if they didn't have much to begin with – as in the case of small-boned women – the density of their bones is further reduced and they are much more fragile and therefore vulnerable to fracture.

We all start losing bone mass from about the age of thirty on, but bone replaces and renews itself, though at a progressively slower rate as the years go by. Collagen, which is the fibrous supporting tissue of bone and skin, gradually disappears, and is only partially replaced. No one knows quite why this happens, although it has been suggested that as we get older we are unable to metabolize protein as efficiently.

Gums and teeth are rarely affected by this bone loss. But if it goes on too long, teeth loosen and infection lodges in the gum pockets around them.

Even though some women are unworried by the effects of the menopause and feel able to put up with the discomforts, it would seem wise to start a course of therapy which would prevent the onset of osteoporosis, particularly if there is already a family history of it. Obviously a balanced diet with perhaps a calcium supplement is important, but a good calcium 'base', to be effective, has to be laid down in childhood. No one is yet sure that calcium additives play a significant part in improvement of the middle-aged skeleton. Therefore, do not put all your faith only in calcium. Women are often advised to drink plenty of milk – skimmed milk is fine if you are worried about weight as it has the same amount of calcium as full-cream milk. Eat yogurt, cheese, tinned tuna, salmon and sardines (again if you have a weight problem, in brine rather than oil), oysters if you can afford them, herrings or mackerel if you can't, and green vegetables like broccoli. Spinach is not, despite its rich source of calcium and iron, because it contains oxalic acid which has the reverse effect upon calcium absorption. Do remember that calcium is not as effective as HRT in stoppping bone loss.

Exercise may be important in arresting the progress of osteoporosis. People who take hard, regular exercise have more bone mass than the slobs among us, but it appears to be the gravity-defying exercises that are more useful than ones such as swimming. Gravity-defying exercise, of course, means running, jogging, tennis, squash – anything that pulls away from gravity. Swimming is good, of course, and keeps the muscles toned without undue strain on the skeleton (which is a factor if you have suffered from a slipped disc or torn a cartilage in your knee) but doesn't seem to have much effect on bone mass in the spine or hip.

If you find it difficult to motivate yourself, try to make a point of tuning in to an exercise programme on television, or join a gym, or simply block off half an hour a day, like a business appointment, and walk briskly, come rain or shine. It's worth it not to end up crippled.

For people who worry about osteoporosis before there are outward signs (and it can creep up on you silently and only show itself when some of the harm has already been done), there are now bone scans available which measure bone mass. They have low radiation doses. These new machines can detect small bone loss before one reaches the risky porous period when fractures are frequent. Unfortunately, they are not available at NHS clinics, but more and more private clinics concentrating on osteoporosis are equipping themselves with them, and if you are one of the women in the high risk group it is worth trying to afford the £150–£200 such a test costs. Because we have a health service it does seem unfair to have to find the money for such tests, but until the NHS is able to fund new, sophisticated equipment we have to rely on the private sector to supply the test. But look at it this way: give up your holiday or a new outfit and you can afford early treatment for a disease that could make the rest of your life a misery.

10
Other problems helped by HRT

HYSTERECTOMY

WOMEN WHO ARRIVE at the menopause latest in life – past the age of fifty – may have less trouble than women who have had either a very early natural menopause or those who had a complete hysterectomy (including removal of the ovaries). For women at the other end of the spectrum, however, and for those who have complete hysterectomies it can be a very different story. One patient, Nadia Rosen, arrived at the Amarant Clinic in a very distressed state:

'I'd always had trouble with my periods and I would pass out in the street from the pain. I was always told it would "clear up" but it didn't until much later. Then I developed cysts on my ovaries. I had three children but my last pregnancy was difficult, landing me in hospital for five and a half months. I haemorrhaged badly after the baby was born and it was decided to give me a complete hysterectomy. Then my problems really started!'

Now an attractive woman of thirty-eight she can laugh

about the situation, but at the time it was no joke. Three days after her hysterectomy, aged twenty-eight, which included the removal of the ovaries, she started to have such heavy night sweats that her bedclothes and nightdress were sopping wet. Wired up to drips and catheters she couldn't reach the window to open it and the night nurse was a dragon who terrified her.

'Some time later I noticed my hair was going grey and my skin was dried up. I tottered to the doctor and he said "Well, of course, after a hysterectomy the ageing process speeds up." I was twenty-eight! I began to get hot flushes and severe water retention. In the morning my feet were so swollen I couldn't put them to the floor without pain. My doctor put me on stronger and stronger diuretics to get rid of the water. I felt terrible. I didn't sleep properly – I used to drop off about 5.30 a.m. and had to be wakened to take the children to school. I was always in a foul temper – I simply put my coat on over my nightdress, warned them not to speak to me, and crawled back to bed as soon as I'd dropped them off. I was evil. I had such mood swings that if I hadn't been a brilliant actress I would be divorced by now. I wasn't interested in sex. I could put up with it as long as I had a book to read and an apple to chew, but as far as enjoyment was concerned, zilch. Yet I'm crazy about my husband – he's wonderful.

'Finally a friend told me I may be damaging myself. "Very high doses of diuretics make your kidneys work harder", she told me. She mentioned the Amarant Trust and I went along, and in a fortnight, I felt a million per cent better. My husband said I even smelt better.'

The happy end to this story is that Nadia has lost all the menopausal symptoms; she sleeps better and she looks wonderful. Her hair, with the low-lights she had put in, looks thick and lustrous and very glamorous. 'At one time,' said Nadia 'I was so depressed by the way I felt and how I looked that I was considering cosmetic surgery. Now I don't need it. I look ten years younger and feel twenty.' Three months ago she started to feel low once more and returned to the Amarant Clinic, where she was monitored and checked all over again, and her HRT dosage adjusted, so that she now feels wonderful again.

The point of this story is that no woman's hormonal pattern is the same, nor does it remain static but with careful checking, the distressing after-effects of the menopause, particularly an artificial menopause brought on by hysterectomy, can be eradicated and the quality of life improved.

PREMATURE MENOPAUSE

In cases where ovaries don't function properly, and the chances of becoming pregnant are reduced, hormone replacement therapy can help alleviate the symptoms which are akin to a premature menopause. They cannot, of course, make women without effective ovaries produce the eggs necessary for fertilization and pregnancy.

One woman, who we shall call Sandra, says that for a long time she did not realize she was infertile.

'I used to have periods only about once every six weeks, but thought nothing of it. Then I had mumps when I was eighteen, and I didn't seem to notice I had not menstruated for six months. Not long afterwards I went on to The Pill.'

At twenty she stopped the Pill and started to have problems with very infrequent periods, she felt constantly tired, and friends at work teased her she was going through the menopause when she had sudden hot flushes. Naturally she consulted her doctor, but her GP shrugged it off saying that in gynaecological matters nothing was 'normal'.

Soon afterwards Sandra got married and began to try for a family, but when by the age of twenty-six she had failed to get pregnant she assumed it was simply bad luck or timing. She became very depressed and would cry in the shower as she got ready for work in the morning. She thought her skin looked old, and her hair lank. Sex was difficult. 'I doubt if we had sex three times in a year. I thought it was because I had gone off my husband.'

She went to her doctor again, asking to be referred to the local hospital for a proper check-up. When she returned to her GP for the results, expecting to be told to take her temperature to discover when she ovulated, or some such simple technique, she was devasted to be told, 'Your ovaries aren't functioning'.

David, her husband was a tower of strength, but Sandra felt overwhelmed:

'The hospital had said I probably needed extra hormones, and because my sister-in-law was being treated at King's for

endometriosis and knew about the work being done there, I plagued my doctor to give me a letter to their specialists.

'I was given an ovarian biopsy, and it was confirmed that I had the ovaries of a fifty-year-old woman, and in all probability the mumps at eighteen had caused the ovarian failure. I knew mumps affected boys, but I had no idea it could have this sort of effect on women.

'They put me on HRT and I am grateful as it has removed some of the physical discomfort. I don't wake up every morning crying, and the hot flushes and the constant tiredness have gone because I can get a good night's sleep now that I no longer suffer from night sweats. But it is no compensation for my infertility. I had no lust, no interest in sex although the vaginal dryness has gone. What is the point of sex if it doesn't result in a baby? I know I'm lucky my husband stays with me.'

Her husband had no illusions about her infertility due to the premature menopause and the emotional problems it brings. He simply hoped for improved techniques, or that they could adopt. But Sandra couldn't accept the situation. She had three attempts at a test-tube baby, using eggs donated by her sister, but without luck.

'It was a hassle and a worry for my sister but it has brought us closer together. My mother was good about it but my father has been critical all along. My parents-in-law are formally uncritical but discreetly cold. Both sets of parents are impatient for grand-children.'

The latest update on Sandra's case is that because she feels better and her skin and hair have improved, her morale is better. She has become reconciled to the situation, and she and David have now adopted two small toddlers.

By the age of twenty-nine Margaret Coombes had the skeletal structure and weight of a woman of seventy. She had a stoop, her hair was lank, her nails brittle and broken. By her own account she looked, and felt herself to be, a deeply unattractive woman. She had lived with her boyfriend for several years but sex was unwelcome to her; her only pleasure was in trying to please him.

As a schoolgirl she had had her first period at thirteen, like her friends, but unlike them hers had stopped altogether when she was fifteen. She was isolated and a swot, and sometimes became alarmingly fat. Because she was determined to get the best exam results in her school and a place at university both she and her mother thought that her periods had stopped due to the stress and anxiety of her schoolwork. Her mother took her to a Harley Street specialist who confirmed this was probably the case and recommended more exercise.

She achieved top exam results and a place at Oxford, but even when the pressure was off her periods did not return. Her GP diagnosed an underactive thyroid, which could have accounted, she thought, for the two bouts of extreme obesity in her teens. '*Even now I can't be sure whether it was hormones that drove me on, or real boredom with frivolous girlish interests.*' But Margaret then found her concentration going, her hair was thin and lustreless, she had brittle fingernails and she started to get panic attacks and bouts of profuse sweating.

Her older sister, a doctor, dismissed Margaret as neurotic, and Margaret, now a university lecturer, was not in a fit state to argue. Eventually, at twenty-nine, she took herself off to a GP again who fortunately arranged for her to have a biopsy. It was then discovered she had complete ovarian failure.

> *'My doctor reluctantly gave me a letter to a special clinic where I had a bone scan. My bones were very low in calcium: lack of oestrogen may have accounted for the condition of my hair and nails. I was put on HRT and within a week I started to feel better. My hair and nails dramatically improved. Even my bones have been "saved". I don't know whether my incipient stoop was due to misery and low morale or the beginnings of a genuine dowager's hump, but at any rate I can stand up straight now.'*

Her childlessness is the source of great anguish. She says she doesn't feel a 'real woman' but as compensation she has developed a new physical closeness with her boyfriend.

> *'For the first time we are lovers — before sex was never a pleasure shared; I endured it for Peter's sake but now I feel interested in sex and lubricate naturally. I can't accept my infertility and am pursuing the idea of a donated egg. My sister seems to have been jolted out of her hostility — she thought my catalogue of disorders was merely an attempt to gain attention and she warned me off HRT as being "dangerous". But now she has seen the improvement and is genuinely sympathetic. She has offered to donate one of her eggs.*
>
> *'All the family rows about my greed and weight. All those indifferent doctors we consulted. They either did not listen or*

didn't know that teenagers without periods are not necessarily tiresome swots. To think I was nearly thirty before it was discovered just what was wrong with me!'

Margaret doesn't see HRT as a cure for something she had – it won't do anything to cure her childlessness, *'but it has stopped me from being a hunched up old lady at thirty-five, and I feel and look so much better.'*

SKIN

Many women report that as they begin the menopause they develop a horrible creeping feeling under their skin, like thousands of insects crawling about. This is called formication. Doctors can't explain it – again, we need more research – but HRT definitely relieves it.

Other women claim their feet and ankles swell and that their fingers feel swollen and stiff. This, too, disappears when they are on a properly balanced HRT routine.

Every woman's body is unique and everyone has a different set of symptoms. But if you take HRT under regular supervision by a menopause specialist they can all be relieved. And as an added bonus your overall health will improve because you are having regular check-ups.

URINARY PROBLEMS

Women, I'm afraid, do seem to have a lot of embarrassing and tiresome problems to cope with, which are due entirely to our biology. If we weren't made to have babies we wouldn't have years of periods or several years of menopausal symptoms, each with their complications and difficulties. Love-making wouldn't be affected by a drying, shrinking vagina, and going to the loo to pass water wouldn't sometimes be accompanied by pain and irritation.

The urethra, which is the small tube into the bladder through which urine is excreted, is partly affected by the menopause, just as the vagina is. Lined with a similar membrane, it dries, becomes less efficient, and the bladder loses some of its control. Sometimes it is necessary to get up during the night to relieve the fullness and the pressure in the bladder and if this happens too often sleep is disturbed with the result that we are tired and ratty in the morning. Worst of all is the difficulty of retaining total control when coughing, sneezing or even running for a bus. 'Stress incontinence' it is called, and women are ashamed of the involuntary wetting of their pants, apart from its discomfort.

This isn't only due to the menopause of course. There is a loss of muscle tone due to sedentary work; often childbirth, particularly if there have been several babies and you weren't totally conscientious about post-natal exercises, will have stretched this area. As will sheer wear and tear, since however hard we try to keep ourselves in good repair, some parts of the body are going to wear out just like metal fatigue in a plane after many take-offs and landings.

Fortunately, HRT can help with the lubrication problems. The natural secretions are slightly acid, which is normally hostile to germs, so that when these secretions dry up there is a greater tendency to pick up infections. Many women find they suffer bouts of cystitis (an inflammation of the urinary bladder) around the time of the menopause before they start a course of HRT. However, once the therapy is started the dryness disappears and an improvement is almost always noticed, sometimes within as little as a week.

There are also things you can do to improve muscle tone if you find that a sudden cough produces that leak. One of the simplest manoeuvres is to interrupt the stream in the middle of a pee. Squeeze the muscles and turn off the tap. Then relax and continue. If you do this every time you go to the loo you will find you gain firmer control. This internal tightening and relaxing of the muscles is an invisible exercise you can do anywhere: whilst watching television, waiting for a bus, chatting at a party. No one will notice but you will probably be more aware of your own posture.

Another exercise involves lying flat on the floor, making sure your lower back is in contact with the floor to avoid back strain, and lifting your pelvis off the floor by contracting the muscles. You should then hold it there for a count of four. Aim for at least fifteen pelvic lifts to begin with and build up to fifty. You'll strengthen your back muscles too!

If you are seriously overweight, make another attempt to lose some poundage, because obesity exacerbates the problem. And cut down on smoking if this has caused a 'smoker's cough' or recurrent bronchitis.

11
Looking good, feeling fit

LEST THE DREADED word 'vanity' pass our lips, let's throw out once and for all the assumption that if you bother to put your best face forward, take some interest in how you look, you are somehow frivolous and feather-headed, devoid of brain power and incapable of serious thought.

It is a fact that when people are mentally low, they lose interest in their appearance. When they receive help and encouragement an improvement in their mental attitude takes place and they may update their hairstyle, wear prettier, more becoming colours, and experiment with make-up, which is why beauty therapists make regular visits to mental hospitals. They know that once the patients begin to care how they look, their mental condition has improved too.

One of our correspondents wrote:

'I am sixty-three and have just succeeded in finding a doctor who has recommended HRT to me. The benefit has been instantaneous, particularly from the mental point of view. I think that if it had been available in my mother's day she may not have spent her last years in and out of mental institutions.

'Now I have been offered a job and want to make the most of

this new opportunity. I don't want to look like an old harridan, so can you tell me about electrolysis and where can I find out about a genuine face lift.'

Perhaps she is being a little carried away by enthusiasm but her letter does illustrate that feeling better makes one want to look better and take up life again.

When women are going through the menopause it often has a deeply depressing effect upon their attitude to life. 'I'm old, life's over, so why bother to look nice? No one is going to look at me anyway . . .' It's a downward spiral – the less trouble you take, the worse you look, so the more your fears are realized, because who wants to talk to someone with a down-turned mouth, wearing dreary, unflattering clothes who clearly hasn't bothered much with her grooming?

Sometimes, as we bemoan the thickening waist, the grey hairs or the wrinkles that have crept up unannounced, we indulge in oral comfort. 'I'll cheer myself up with a cup of coffee and a biscuit', 'I'll pop into this tea shop for some nice hot buttered scones and a pot of tea', 'I'll treat myself to a box of chocolates'. Treating yourself to consoling little snacks, sinking away from reality and the dreariness of your problems by putting your feet up and watching a television 'soap', all pile on the pounds and suddenly attractive clothes in your size are much harder to come by.

All right, you may be over the first flush of youth but that doesn't mean you have to give in without a fight. Nothing is more pathetic than an older woman trying to pretend she's still a teenager, but what we're talking about is taking care of ourselves – mind and body. We're into the age of glamorous older women now, so it can be done. Mrs Thatcher, Miriam

Stoppard, Joan Collins, Jane Fonda, Kate O'Mara, Jill Gascoine, Edna O'Brien, Shirley Maclaine, Sian Phillips, Gayle Hunnicut . . . the list of really attractive women who are well into middle age and beyond is endless. And they are not women with nothing better to do than loll around at health farms being massaged and cossetted, painted and powdered. Most have exhausting jobs as well as families, which could be one of the keys to it all.

Anyone busy, particularly anyone in the public eye, *has* to work out a routine that ensures they look good all the time, or the media, with their cruel cameras and assassinating articles, pounce mercilessly. Career women can't afford to let up either, because once your grooming slips it is assumed your grasp on the job is slipping too.

One of the best investments for an older woman – apart from a clued-up, sympathetic GP – is a ruthlessly, revealingly honest, magnifying mirror. Some people are lucky enough to have magnificent sight all their lives, but most of us, as we get older, become long-sighted and squinting in an ordinary dressing-table mirror is not going to show you the stray superfluous hairs furring the outline of chin and upper lip, or the pathetic smudges where your make-up has been applied with less than accurate targeting, particularly if you wear eye make-up, or the thread veins on cheeks which your misty eyes saw simply as healthy colour. Besides, eye make-up, which should be discreet and subtle unless you are a punk, can't be applied whilst you are wearing specs; you *need* a magnifying glass to put it on properly.

A good magnifying mirror that gives a frank close-up without distortion, and is large enough to have a good old peer at your skin, is not cheap – anything from £25–70 depending on size and framing. A man's good shaving mirror is probably the cheapest, but often they have to be fixed to the wall. Some stores sell a framed mirror with a large hook as a stand which makes it portable but which will also sling round your neck so that you can move to the best light, leaving your hands free. Test them out until you find one that frightens the wits out of you in close-up and buy that – it will be your best friend.

Above all, budget for money to spend entirely on yourself. It is *not* selfish. It need not be a lot, but if you don't have any money to invest in your appearance you're never going to be able to afford to keep your hair style up to date, the essential jar of moisturizer and handcream, and the spirit-lifting quality of a good bottle of scent. Now is the time to put yourself first. It pays off because people take you at your own valuation. A smart, confident, attractive woman is treated accordingly. Someone overweight, apologetic and put together with a clumsy hand is overlooked and ignored. Let the cushions and carpet wait, if necessary, until next year.

FIGURING IT OUT

Let's start with your figure because, if that is trim, so much else falls into place. If you are overweight you tend to waddle rather than walk, your back rounds with pads of fat over the shoulder blades, the upper arms puff so that you have to choose sleeve styles carefully, and the stomach can't be held in flat no matter how hard you try. Undressed, the body looks as quilted and spongy as cottage cheese. You also breathe less freely which cuts down the oxygen supply to the blood. The neck thickens, chins disappear, ankles swell . . . shall we go on? Or does it sound enough of a horror story to make you realize that letting the pounds build up is not only ageing and debilitating but makes the search for becoming clothes frustrating and time-consuming?

You can always do something about your weight, even if you're never going to achieve – and may not want to – the emaciated shape of a flat-chested model girl. Some of us may have a body type that will always look a little solid, or a large frame, and you can't change this however much you diet or exercise, because bone size and genetics will always win. But there is a point where the body's natural weight is exceeded to the extent that you are toting around a lot of unnecessary luggage.

Check your weight against the height-and-weight tables printed below. If you are over the top limit (and as you can see there is a lot of leeway) give yourself a constructive fright by weighing a sackful of potatoes that equals the amount by which you are over the limit. Then imagine carrying that in a shopping bag day in, day out, upstairs and downstairs, in fact everywhere. You'd feel tired and puffed, wouldn't you? That's precisely what happens to your body – heart and lungs become strained and, like anything that is constantly tired, cease to function efficiently.

Losing weight is not a question of racing for the nearest diet fad and being self-disciplined for a couple of weeks. It needs a new lifestyle, a determination to equate the food going in with the energy going out, which, yes, means eating less and exercising more. If it all sounds rather depressing, let

How much should you weigh for your height?			
Height	Small frame	Medium frame	Large frame
ft in	st lb	st lb	st lb
4 10	6 11	7 3	7 13
4 11	6 13	7 6	8 2
5 0	7 2	7 9	8 5
5 1	7 5	7 12	8 8
5 2	7 8	8 1	8 11
5 3	7 11	8 4	9 0
5 4	8 0	8 7	9 3
5 5	8 4	8 11	9 7
5 6	8 6	9 1	9 11
5 7	8 10	9 5	10 1
5 8	9 0	9 9	10 5
5 9	9 4	9 13	10 9
5 10	9 9	10 3	11 0
5 11	9 13	10 7	11 4
6 0	10 5	10 11	11 9

(NB: To convert into metric one inch is approximately 2.54 cm, 2.2lb is approximately 1 kg.

us cheer you up by making a promise: you *will* feel better and you most certainly *will* look better.

The hard part is just getting started on a bit more exercise, when you have been used to taking a bus or driving the car to your various destinations. The mental sloth is harder to overcome than the physical reluctance. Once you have forced yourself into doing something more energetic you somehow seem to acquire more mental energy; you have climbed the barrier between exercising and not exercising. The first week or two are the hardest. Your muscles are slack and it seems hard work to move easily, but keep at it – ten minutes a day is all it takes to help you gradually loosen up and everyone can spare that. Just keep going, working a little bit harder each time and don't fall back just because you miss a day and think 'oh that's it'. *Perseverance pays.*

Walk more, swim more – both are the best and simplest exercises – or join a gym class if you need encouragement from other women. One woman acquired a dog that had to be taken for daily walks and she was surprised to find at the end of a month she had lost 7lb without noticing it, and without dieting. If she had eaten just a bit less, smaller portions than usual, nothing between meals, kept a careful eye on puddings, sweets, cakes and between-meal snacks, she would have lost another 7lb.

Simple exercise like walking the dog, as long as it is a brisk walk and not a slow amble, speeds up the circulation which has good results throughout the body. Look at people returning from playing tennis or cycling and their complexions positively glow. Instead of tiring you out, moderate exercise actually tops up your energy so that you feel more alert, brisker. It also makes your metabolism work better so that the food you do eat is used as energy, not laid down as fat.

Exercise, if you haven't been very energetic for a long time, must be done slowly to begin with. Hunters that have been turned out for the summer are *walked* to tone up their muscles for a couple of weeks before they are gently trotted, then cantered and finally galloped – a process that takes four to six weeks before they are ready for the hunting field. A stiffened or flabby body must not be forced into a programme that would floor a boxer – do gentle stretching exercises to begin with, or go to yoga classes until you've firmed the flab and oiled the joints.

One point to make is that walking or running should not be done too briskly without wearing shoes with cushioned rubber soles. Thin, leather-soled shoes jar the spine too much and your virtuous exercise could end up doing more harm than good. They don't have to be as conspicuous as trainers, although American women who look after their appearance walk to work in business suits and training shoes and carry their smart shoes in their briefcases!

YOU ARE WHAT YOU EAT

By now those words are a cliché, but like many clichés they have a lot of truth. In this country it would be very difficult to become undernourished even if you existed on junk food, but a varied, well-thought-out diet keeps the body in good nick. Just as a high-performance car won't run on two-star fuel, if you want the best from your body – healing and repair of bones and tissue, a defence armoury to repel and vanquish invading germs, general maintenance for efficient function, and an attacking force so that if at some stage you are unlucky enough to be struck by a serious disease you are more able to marshal reserves and fight back – then you must give some intelligent thought to what you're putting in the tank.

It is generally agreed by doctors and nutrition experts that the 'Western diet', the one we in Britain eat, is not as healthy as the diet of Japanese, Chinese, Indians and Mexicans (providing they get enough to eat) because we rely heavily on meat, and meat has too much fat for our health – even lean meat still contains 'invisible' fat. The countries mentioned above eat more rice, beans and lentils, which are mainly all carbohydrates and protein, and contain little or no fat. Our diet is also rich in milk, butter and dairy products, and although they contain calcium, vitamins, and other essential elements, they too, like meat, contain high proportions of fat. The answer is to switch to skimmed milk, yogurts, low-fat cheeses and butter substitutes. Avoid fried and roasted foods. Substitute fish or lentils for some of your current meat meals. Bake potatoes in their jackets or mash them with a little skimmed milk; don't toss vegetables in butter as a matter of course. Reconsider some of your cooking habits to see if unwittingly you are adding more fat than you thought.

It is not easy to overcome a lifetime of bad eating habits. You don't want to make meals a misery for yourself, or any good resolutions will be quickly ditched, but there are certain simple things you can do which will trim off little fattening extras that all add up. Study food labels to find out if, say, a tin of baked beans contains unnecessary sugar. Labelling has got much better in supermarkets these days, so never shop without your specs if you can't read without them.

Ideally, take as much as you can of your diet in raw, fresh foods so that you avoid preservatives, smoked, pickled or highly salted foods and various unnecessary additives. Aim for fifty per cent, if possible, snacking on scrubbed fresh vegetables like celery, peppers, carrots, string beans; steam or grill as much as possible – vegetables look and taste better lightly steamed, and the juices can be used to make light sauces, soup stock or gravy.

Grilling extracts fat, which cuts down the calories and cholesterol so use the grill pan rather than the frying pan. If you've been used to plates piled high with helpings of meat, thickened gravies, roast potatoes and soggy green vegetables you have to re-train your palate to the lighter, simple fare. It won't be easy at first, but it pays off in terms of better health and better shape. If iron resolve rails and you indulge in a guilty bout of bingeing, don't give up. Start again. You can't undo a lifetime's habits in five minutes, so be kind to yourself. Don't despair.

Cut back on sugar – don't believe honey is less fattening. All sugars – and that includes fructose, the fruit sugars, are roughly equivalent in calories. If you must have sugar in tea or coffee use the sugar substitutes but remember whilst you go on sweetening your drinks, you will never wean your taste buds away from the flavour. It is possible to learn to like things that are less sweet, less salty, less fatty. If you don't believe that statement think back to the foods you disliked as a child; many of them you eat with relish now have been an acquired taste.

Biscuits, cakes, sweets and chocolate should be banned altogether if you are serious about altering your eating habits, but it would be inhuman to pass up the occasional treat. Indeed, sometimes relaxing an iron discipline strengthens your determination when you go back to the regimen; you feel you are in control.

Experiment with various herbal teas until you find a couple that you find pleasing enough to substitute, at least sometimes, for tea and coffee. Cut down alcohol, never more than three, preferably two, small glasses of wine or its equivalent a day, and try to have one or two alcohol-free days each week. Fortunately because of the concern over alcohol-related disease and the laws on drinking and driving, manufacturers and brewers have been stimulated into producing a wide range of low-alcohol or alcohol-free drinks, and some are quite acceptable substitutes for wine and spirits.

This book isn't about dieting – there must be hundreds on the subject – but it is about looking after yourself so that you are fit enough to enjoy life, and if you are overweight then, sorry, you are not fit.

If you feel indignantly virtuous about how little you eat, and unjustly maligned because you still put on weight, keep a private diary for a month or everything that passes your lips. Don't guess, weigh things. A piece of bread you think is half an ounce may easily weigh two; you forget how many cups of tea you have drunk with full-cream milk and sugar; the second biscuit you took, the family 'left-overs' you finished off behind the scenes in the kitchen because you 'can't bear to waste food'. It is better to throw away the spoonful of roast potatoes, the lonely slice of cake, than have them padding out your hips. The 'bottom line' at the end of the day will astonish you.

Write down how much activity you took, better still buy or borrow a pedometer. You will probably be ruefully surprised at how unbalanced your food intake is with your energy output, and what isn't used up in fuelling activity doesn't drain harmlessly away; it is stored all over the body until you look as though you're permanently clad in a duvet!

SKINCARE

Skin dries out as it is gradually weathered over the years by wind, sun – particularly sun – and atmospheric pollution, and begins to look more like crêpe paper, particularly if it hasn't been protected by a moisturizer.

Under the surface of the skin there is a supporting network of collagen fibres, a bit like mattress springs. Collagen is also part of the framework of bone so, like bone, the collagen in skin is also affected by the menopause. With a decrease in the body's own hormonal activity, bone loss accelerates so that the skeleton becomes more porous and fragile, and skin likewise thins, the supporting mattress of collagen fibres begins to sag like an old bed.

Any woman put on hormone therapy notices a distinct improvement in her skin after about six month's treatment. It won't miraculously eradicate wrinkles, but it will make the skin appear plumper, moister, more youthful, as if a steam iron has been run over it. If this internal treatment is combined with more oxygen in the bloodstream due to exercise, coupled with a well-balanced diet, and simple skincare, you can look a great deal younger. Perhaps this is why some people equate HRT with narcissism or vanity; they have a grudge against other women looking good, or as they put it, 'flying in the face of Nature'.

Very little of what you apply to the skin can sink in – the skin is meant to prevent that. But a daily routine of cleansing, toning, nourishing can keep the outer layer clean and moist so that it looks better. Even if you don't use make-up, cleansing the skin thoroughly is a good idea because of the amount of dirt and pollution in the atmosphere, particularly if you live in a city. Cream or lotions are kinder to a dry, older skin than soap and water, and they are more effective in removing the remains of make-up at the end of the day, since they emulsify with the oils in the cosmetics, which soap and water don't. It makes sense when you consider that beauty-preparation manufacturers spend a great deal of money researching the lasting qualities of their foundation preparations. Something they claim will stay on all day is not going to be removed completely with a soapy flannel.

Toning is done by whisking over the face and neck a cotton-wool ball or a tissue sprinkled with a slightly astringent lotion that effectively removes the last of the cleanser, and helps to keep a fine texture.

Nourishing is something of a misnomer because the only thing that actually 'nourishes' the skin is the bloodstream, but smoothing a film of moisturizing cream over the skin is like a fine waterproof layer: it reduces the loss of water without which no skin can look good. Daily moisturizers, backed up by a heavier, richer night cream helps to prevent drying. Of course, many companies will spend lots of advertising pounds on making you believe that fancy jars and packaging are all part of the do-gooding, but there are many inexpensive preparations which are just as effective. The point is to treat your skin kindly. Some women have marvellously fine skins that they are fortunately able to retain all their lives, but ordinary complexions reveal signs of wear and tear if they don't have a modicum of protection.

If you look at a racehorse in the paddock it is groomed to perfection; its coat is burnished to a high gloss, its hooves are oiled and 'manicured', its mane gleams and there isn't an ounce of superfluous weight. It has been fed well, exercised thoroughly and checked out regularly by its doctor, the veterinary surgeon. Compare it with a turned-out horse in a field. The unbrushed coat is dull and dirty, the diet of grass is adequate but not necessarily of high quality, and there is not the incentive to gallop and do a measured trot round the field. Most horses, left to themselves, graze gently and just have a little canter to break the monotony. The parallel with humans is obvious. An intelligent diet, a variety of interests, attention to health, and good grooming will keep us in competitive shape.

HAIR AND MAKE-UP

The psychological effect of looking attractive and up to date should not be underestimated. A woman who attracts admiration and appraising looks has more confidence, more pleasure in being herself, so don't let anyone persuade you that once you are into the menopause you lose all allure.

It is all too easy to get into a rut and not notice you've hung on to the same hairstyle you had in your twenties. At the other extreme some women don't want to be bothered with looking after themselves and go in for one of those short over-curly perms which they consider saves time and trouble. Perhaps it does – and it shows. A short, frizzy halo seems to be the hallmark of older women, regardless of their face shape or lifestyle.

The best insurance scheme is to put your head literally into the hands of a good hairdresser. If you can't afford to spend a lot, have it professionally re-styled once or twice a year, and learn to shampoo and set it yourself in a fashionable style between visits. Don't go to a good hairdresser and tell him or her how you want it done; that's keeping a dog and barking yourself. You're paying for an objective, expert view on a contemporary style to suit you, so keep an open mind until you've tried a new style. If after a short trial it feels uncomfortable and not 'you', no harm is done – you can change it.

A sobering lesson can be learned from one very well-known writer, who shall be anonymous, who had a professional 'make-over' for a Sunday newspaper feature. She looked wonderful and went home excited and treading on air. Her husband and teenage children were appalled. This wasn't the dumpy, frumpy mum they were used to. They felt threatened, her husband was afraid other men would be attracted. They nagged so much she reverted to her previous dull hairstyle and faded back into the wallpaper.

Tinting and colouring is not to be considered if you are short of money because it needs to be done well. Expert colourists will blend the professional tints and dyes to suit individuals. If it is done amateurishly the shades aren't adapted to your changing skintones and can look harsh and even more ageing. The contrast between unbelievable blonde hair that looks good on a Marilyn Monroe looks somehow pathetic on a woman over fifty. Some over-the-counter do-it-yourself colour rinses are effective, particularly if your own natural colour has simply faded a bit and needs a lift or if it has gone that rather unbecoming pepper-and-salt grey. They are not permanent so, again, it is worth experimenting to see what they do for you. But avoid 'red' and 'black' – both can look hard.

As we've said before, this book isn't primarily about diet and beauty, but if you look good you feel good and a lift to the morale is vital to anyone. Make-up is an expert's ball-game, but most stores will have sales assistants who have some training in the choice and use of their products; but remember they are there to *sell*, so don't be dragooned into buying a lot of unsuitable preparations that might do well in a laser-lit disco but have little relationship to your persona.

Make-up is another area where a trained, independent expert can be invaluable. Look for a beauty shop in your town. Barbara Daly, one of the world's cleverest make-up artists (responsible for Princess Diana's wedding day make-up, in demand by enough 'royals' and celebrities to put *Who's Who* in the shade) has evolved a simple range of make-up for the Body Shop chain under her 'Colourings' label, These are inexpensive and straightforward, and co-ordinated into a range for different skin types. Most Colourings assistants receive training to help with advice, but Barbara, ever prag-matic, has also produced an instructional video on how make-up should be applied to look soft and natural – it costs £9.94 from the Body Shop and selected branches of W. H. Smith. If you fear your make-up techniques are rusty and out of date, you might find it helpful. And, since it demonstrates methods, it is just as relevant to other brands of cosmetics. In any case, most of us can do with a refresher course now and then.

Make-up 'looks' and shades change with fashion and nothing looks more dated than hanging on to sparkly, vibr-ant blue eyeshadow applied with a trowel when everyone else is subtly shadowed with a hint of grey or brown. If you believe 'a rose is a rose is a rose' and that there isn't much you can do with lipstick and powder, try glancing at old photograph albums! Snapshots taken as little as ten years ago have a dated quality and if you don't change – ideas as well as looks – you have that set frozen-in-aspic quality like the characters in a period play.

There is no need to be a slavish follower of fashion. Your own style and comfort determine how you want to look, but you need to make adjustments to your style, to move on a little. If you're afraid of getting it wrong, keep abreast of the changes in contemporary looks by checking out the fashion and beauty pages of some of the smarter women's magazines from time to time.

And do get an honest second opinion on your efforts.

12

For men

WHAT ARE YOU going to do about your partner? Here she is, nice home, loving husband, possibly less money worries than you had when you were first married, children, if any, leading their own lives. Why does she seem so cross and irritable with you? Why only the other day when you came home it was obvious she had been crying.

She's gone off sex too. She doesn't seem to want you any more. Says 'it hurts', or she's tired. Sometimes when you attempt to touch her at night she feels soaking wet. Not the best way to make love is it, to someone who has a face like a wet week, complains and moans all the time, won't let you touch her. Even during the day she sometimes looks hot and bothered.

Can't be anything medically wrong with her. You made her see the doctor not long ago and he said there was nothing really the matter. Perhaps she needs a holiday . . .

Perhaps there's someone else? She certainly seems to toss and turn a lot at night, perhaps she has a guilty conscience. Wakes you up sometimes too. Doesn't she realize that you *need* your sleep?

No, it can't be another man. She's let herself go and that's not a sign of an illicit romance. But her hair doesn't seem so pretty these days, and her skin looks somehow grey. Oh well, we're both getting old. But I wish she'd buck up a bit. I'm beginning to dread coming home after work in case I get my head bitten off . . .

Those actual words may not be running through your head but unless you are one of those amazingly understanding men who know something about women's biology you have probably thought something along those lines in your bewilderment at the change in your wife or partner.

It can't be easy to find yourself living with someone who seems to have turned into a perfect stranger – and sometimes not a very pleasant stranger at that. If it is any comfort, she is probably just as bothered and bewildered as you are. You'd think women would know all about how their bodies work and the interlink between physical and psychological symptoms. But many don't.

It is really very simple but not explained often enough. And even today, despite every subject under the sun seemingly being discussed fully and frankly on television, no one seems to get to grips with the problem of the menopause. You wouldn't think – from the secrecy that surrounds it – it affects millions of people every year. It might happen to women but it affects their friends and families, too, and chiefly, of course, you.

Everyone knows that because we are all living a lot longer, we are an ageing society – but old age in women is almost always depicted as some decrepit old dear terrified of crossing the road. Its ludicrous when you think about it. Imagine someone having the temerity to offer to guide Mrs Thatcher across a zebra crossing! Yet she's in her mid-sixties. Imagine expecting Katie Boyle, Joan Collins or Dr Miriam Stoppard to sit sipping Horlicks in an armchair whilst watching something mindless on television before toddling off to an early bed!

Older men are sometimes ridiculed by younger ones, but not as hurtfully as women are. Women are called 'old bags' and other wounding names to describe those who are past the last flush of youth; in films and television they are invariably portrayed as fat and fraying at the edges whenever a late middle-aged female character is called for. Meek and pathetic on some occasions or loud and aggressive on others.

The menopause, or the 'change', which in all probability your wife is going through right now, is often treated as a joke or an embarrassment by men. It shouldn't be. It is her reaction to the run-down in her body's reproductive function. Luckily for men, they don't suffer the same sudden close down. They go on being fertile. For women, however, there's a redundancy programme in progress as some departments of the works are made obsolete. Like any change-over there are going to be some hiccups. The hormones in your wife's body aren't quite as obedient as the brain would like. Some are going to go on producing, refusing to accept notice; whilst others will be only too grateful to shut down and put their feet up. One minute your partner's feet are cold, the next she is throwing off the bedclothes and changing her nightdress. If left to simply get on with it, it will be some time before everything settles down, perhaps as long as *five years*.

Fortunately, things can be brought under control quite quickly. We know that the chief hormone controlling all the current changes in your wife's body is oestrogen, but as the menopause progresses the supplies of this substance diminish. And because the body is no longer concerned with making babies, the vagina begins to dry up. As it dries it shrinks and thins, even changes shape. When you attempt intercourse there is no natural lubrication and the thin walls can easily get damaged by your movement. They tear and break, and infection can develop.

Natural oestrogen, however, can be made outside the body, in a laboratory, and this will quickly restore the lubrication and reduce or banish altogether the daytime hot flushes and the nighttime sweats. As she begins to feel better, her moods will disappear. She gets back her old enjoyment of life, and her energy. Her skin and hair may also improve. The dryness and lack-lustreness you noticed are not due to self-neglect but to a genuine breakdown in the underpinning of the skin.

A woman needs two female hormones to make the treatment medically safe. Your wife may, as a result, return to having a light monthly bleed, similar to a period but this isn't always so, and nor does it mean she can get pregnant again.

If your wife or partner has been going through this difficult time you can be of enormous help to her. First of all you must show her you realize her mood swings are nothing to do with you, but are merely due to a temporary hormonal imbalance. Be extra loving and reassuring during this time. One of our correspondents said she would have felt so much better if her husband had just put his arm round her, given her a cuddle, instead of making her feel in solitary confinement inside a prison of baffling emotions.

Secondly, encourage her to see her doctor. Go with her if you can, as moral support, because some doctors are still inclined to treat menopausal symptoms as something you put up with like a passing bout of indigestion, and that they usually only affect hypochondriacs. There *is* something that can be done for your wife and if her GP is disinclined to help her she must ask to be referred to a menopause clinic or a gynaecologist. Don't let the doctor fob you off with tranquillizers or anti-depressants. In the short term these may be necessary but they can only give temporary relief.

Once she gets to a clinic she may have a series of tests to determine what kind of treatment she needs, and will be given a prescription. Often a letter will be written to her GP outlining the treatment suggested so that he can carry on with the prescription. He may be willing to monitor her progress. Each woman is different and sometimes the dose needs minor adjusting.

Not only will she return to 'normal' very shortly, but the treatment will also protect against bone loss. Once she is taking oestrogen regularly there is a reduced likelihood of your wife risking the fractures that bedevil many women after their fifties, some of them proving fatal. Nor will she be quite so liable to heart attacks and strokes. When the benefits are so great, and the drawbacks so small, there seems little point in hesitating, does there?

And it may save your marriage.

Case histories

June McKay

'I AM ASHAMED TO SAY that I used to think the menopause was a lot of fuss about nothing. I thought women should take their ageing gracefully and enjoy it. The crumbly, defeated women that I met I regarded as feeble, lost without their children at home, weary of their husbands or stuck in jobs which they considered demeaning.'

June McKay is a tall, attractive woman with fair hair and the kind of skin which always looks tanned. She has never lost a no-nonsense Lancashire accent even though she has lived in stockbroker Surrey since her husband's work took them south fifteen years ago. 'I knew all about the menopause and one of the things I knew was that it would never affect me.'

When it did affect her she was, she says, a disaster to live with. 'I was completely unable to sleep . . . just lay there sweating and panicking, panicking and sweating. My heart thumped away and I had pools of sweat in my nightclothes and in the bedding. Ewan, my husband, was sympathetic but baffled. I realize now just how good he was because he never

got a night's sleep either and I was aggressive and difficult
. . . it was a frightening experience.

'I suppose you can say that it served me right, but I found
my friends and neighbours singularly unsympathetic – they
took my previous attitude that it was a song and dance about
nothing. In fact, it had taken me some time to recognize that
my trouble was the menopause. At first I thought it was a
virus, some sort of fever. I can only describe my GP's
attitude as one of total indifference: he actually laughed at me
and told me not to be so silly.

'I lost not only my confidence and self-respect, but my
concentration too. Some days I felt real hatred for Ewan: it
sounds silly, but I loathed him because he was getting at least
some sleep. I was intolerable company, we weren't getting
asked out any more and I had become the authentic old bag
. . . I see it now although I could see nothing at the time.'

Eventually it was her sister-in-law, not her doctor, who
told her about HRT, and she only knew what she had read in
a woman's magazine. 'If it had not been for her casual reading, I would still be falling apart. In the end, my doctor
prescribed the cream, it wasn't the miracle cure I was half-
expecting, but distinctly better. The night-sweats were mild-
er and my temper improved. Then I converted to the pills
and at once I felt young again.

'I was surprised by the cosmetic advantages as I had not
been told about them. I had spots, which went. My skin was
more supple and my hair got its colour and shine back. When
I think of that doctor smirking at me I feel very angry. I have
tackled him about it since and he says he was never taught
about HRT and regarded it as cranky medicine. But it is not

the memory of his ignorance that upsets me – it's his cruelty.'

Veronica Bain

'I didn't have any sensation of being sterile, but when I asked advice about why my periods had stopped the woman consultant at the hospital told me very bluntly that my ovaries were not functioning and that I could not have children. I was only thirty and I found this a great shock, not the least because I was milling around with so many friends who were pregnant, even surrounded by them at the hospital clinic.'

Veronica Bain is a solicitor. Divorced, she takes a fierce pride in her ability to think and cope for herself. 'I was deeply uneasy about the idea of HRT. It seemed to me to be a masculine device for disposing – one way or another – of troublesome women. I wasn't reassured about the risk of the dreaded C. I found the idea of keeping fit by diet and supplements like vitamins and calcium far more attractive and convincing. Anyway dietary fads are comprehensible, most of medicine is bamboozling.

'I put up with some of the usual physical symptoms: sweats, back ache and so on. But I couldn't bear it when my efficiency in the office was impaired. I was moody and my memory was dreadful: even things that I had said a few minutes before I found myself repeating. My colleagues didn't criticize me but I was painfully aware of my shortcomings.

'I was celibate at this time: I think I was pursuing a grudge against men after the break-up of my marriage. But I was becoming aware that my lack of interest was not the intellectual decision I thought it to be, not feminist hostility but plain lack of libido.

'I almost willed the treatment to fail. But I'm forced to say that the effect was immediate. Within a fortnight I was transformed. Only then did I realize how low I had been – I felt twenty years younger.

'Now I have become a disciple for the cause. It is a mad system that doesn't make the knowledge and the choice available to all women who are in need of help. It is because women's careers are not regarded as serious. It doesn't matter if their continuity of work is broken. If it happened to men they would get sympathy and treatment – you know how important their work is to them.

'I'm eternally grateful that I stumbled on HRT and I have to say I'm grateful for what was intolerable bullying by the hospital doctor. Fortunately he knew what he was talking about.'

Emma Lynn

Emma Lynn, at the age of sixty, is a tall, elegant woman who used to be a fashion buyer, and it shows. Her appearance gives little clue as to her age or her history of bone troubles, which started when her hip was crushed in a road accident twenty-five years ago. She was not worried by the menopause ('In a strange way I enjoyed the warmth of the change – I wallowed quite happily in my sweat!') but she *was* concerned about the effects on her skeleton. That is what took her to King's College Hospital. She had read about their work on HRT in a magazine article.

'Once I had started on first the cream and then the pills my poor legs felt stronger and I felt generally improved. The doctors said that my deterioration had been halted, that my osteoporosis was well advanced but it was holding. I was fortunate that my spine was unaffected. By the way, without being told to expect it, I noticed that my nails – toe-nails in particular – came back to life and my hair got its colour back. If I have a complaint, it's that HRT came too late to work its best, it can't erase that accident all those years ago.

'I've gone back to work – quite a small job but a nice little earner and very good for my self-respect – and I feel ashamed of the misery I've caused my husband. Our sex life had dwindled to almost nothing, although I never did have that trouble with my vagina drying out. I just had no interest and I think Tom was frightened to ask. Now I wouldn't say I was exactly randy but I'm quite willing. I think we have a good sex life now, not as good as ten years ago, but Tom has his own problems on that score: he's ten years older. I enjoy cuddling, whereas before all contact repelled me.

'I regret the two years of misery and I'm angry that my GP was no help at all. HRT seems to me to be wonderful and I am disgusted that it seems to be restricted to women who have the money, the contacts or the push.'

Joan Gingell

Joan Gingell works in a family planning clinic. Nevertheless, it took her a ten-year struggle to get beyond her GP's opposition to HRT.

Joan got to know about HRT through her work and when she started to feel thoroughly ill and miserable ('hot flushes, irritable, revolted by the thought of sex and a husband who was thoroughly fed up with me') she started to do some more reading.

'My GP said HRT was against all his instincts as a Catholic. To interfere with the bodily processes would be "against Nature". He offered me blood-pressure tablets. I waited until he went on holiday and asked his locum. But she said it would 'thicken my uterus'. She muttered audibly under her breath about wretched neurotic women. I was meant to hear.

'I am not that brave a person and hate confrontations but it was the idea of osteoporosis, I think, which firmed me up. My grandmother had shrunk in height and I could see it happening to my mother and to my sister as well. I stood my ground and got my way, but it took ten years.

'I never saw what my doctor said in his letter of referral and I expect that's just as well! At the hospital they simply said I wasn't producing enough natural hormones. The effect on my spirits and my morale were extraordinary and very fast. But most of my optimism I'm saving for the long-term. I am hoping to escape some of the osteoporosis and avoid what is happening to my poor mother.'

Jean Armand

When Jean Armand, at the age of forty-six, went to her GP with 'normal' but extremely unpleasant menopausal symptoms, he told her: 'There's no need to do anything – this is just the way God's chosen to make you.' He did refer her to a gynaecologist, but she said: 'Oh well, God could have thought up a worse way of ending your child-bearing life.'

'I made a serious tactical error', says Jean, 'on a follow-up visit to the GP I told him that I had read about HRT in a women's magazine. He was doubly disdainful – of women who quote remedies they have read about in magazines, and of the treatment itself. I tried the subject on his wife when she was a locum for him and she was openly hostile.

'My sweats were so dreadful that I couldn't work and dreaded going into the office or anywhere in public (Jean is a writer in an advertising agency). My first real flush had occurred at Gatwick Airport, of all places, as we were about to fly out to Greece on holiday. I thought I was going to pass out and my eyes puffed up so that I could hardly see. My husband thought I was throwing a tantrum and told me to relax and breathe deeply. I think he thought I was just going barmy. Now he is very understanding. Actually, we were lucky in one respect: our sex life had not been impaired. I was restless and irritable but I never had the problem of my vagina drying out, like I know other people have.

'I think I would still be suffering my symptoms if my boss had not been so kind. He saw how discomforted I was and pushed me into approaching King's, which he had heard about.' The consultant there relaxed his insistence on a doctor's letter of referral when the problem was explained to him.

'I have been on HRT for six years – I am fifty-three now – and no one will persuade me it's harmful. My sister was taken off HRT at the insistence of her GP. Both my older sisters have started to get obvious curvature of the spine. My mother has suffered dreadfully from osteoporosis and is very stooped. I am sorry for her and pleased for myself to be minimizing the risk.

'I enjoy life, I can work creatively. I am grateful to King's and to my boss. Two other small but important things . . . my hands and hair improved. And definitely my memory. I blame HRT for my extra weight – but then it's good to have something to blame it on!'

Anna Powrie

Anna Powrie was a school bursar but she gave up her job when she convinced herself she was going mad. 'I was always irritable and absent-minded, to a degree which couldn't pass for normal. That would be bad enough in any job but I was doing work which needed at least simple arithmetic and some diplomacy. They must have thought I was a horrible old bag and a bitch . . . because I was!

'I kept bursting into tears. The headmaster joked to me years later that he had thought I had a crush on him. I used to insist everyone else shiver while I sat glowing hot and sweating with the windows wide open. My colleagues were amazingly patient, looking back on it, but David my husband had the worst of it.

'I had virtually given up any domestic duties . . . I could not be bothered to wash or cook, although I still tidied up. I think that was part of my routine and it had a certain therapeutic value. And he must have gone ten years with no real sign of tenderness from me.

'I realized my periods had stopped and that I was showing the symptoms of an unhappy menopause. I asked my GP if he thought this was sensible (he is a friend of my husband's so I was reticent about telling him all the details). He was really very cruel. He laughed and just said I was getting old –

at fifty-two. I remember he gave me some leaflets about Christianity. David was annoyed at that and I went back to say I didn't think Jesus was my problem. He was courteous but obviously annoyed at me pursuing the matter and made me feel I was pestering him. But he did refer me to the hospital and I could not have been more impressed.

'I wasn't treated like a fool. They listened. They did a biopsy and then prescribed a series of pills. Six weeks later I was on an even keel again. The hot flushes disappeared. I actually slept at night. My husband said he thought I was becoming reasonable again. Life became bearable, and then pleasant, and now sometimes even delightful.

'I am fit and competent. David still gets no intercourse but that is more due to his ill health than mine. I fondle him and I can please him but he has a slipped disc, a hernia and a bypass so we are hardly athletic.

'I probably would have retired anyway by now, but I know my menopause brought me out of my job too soon, and it makes me sad that they must remember me as a miserable sort of person. Now I'm out and about and do a lot of voluntary work but it is not the same as doing a professional, salaried job with competence.

'I read that one in five women suffer no real ill-effects from the menopause – but that leaves four-fifths of us who have a grim time. It is ridiculous doctors seem to be untrained or indifferent. I've tried to talk about HRT to GPs I know socially and they smirk and think it is daft.

'I have at least changed my doctor – to a woman. She is fifty, and understands.'

Viv Linklater

'I have come across so many middle-aged women decaying and distressed . . . I used to see it as sexism, allowing them to rot; the attitude that once their childbearing years are over women are not needed any more. Now I think I am more sympathetic towards doctors. I realize that it is not all deliberate cruelty – they are ignorant about so much.'

Viv Linklater is a very successful career woman, a theatrical agent. Forceful, rather alarmingly outspoken and aggressive, she still regards the medical profession as a patriarchy which cares little for the needs of women. It is hard to imagine any GP ignoring her requests for help. At the same time she makes it plain that she is wary of their advice and capable of reading up the medical literature for herself if she really wants to know something.

Nevertheless, it was a full two years after being told that her ovaries were no longer functioning before she started on HRT. For all her belief in patient choice, she feels that she should have been guided towards it more specifically. But she herself had strong reservations – it was her own reading about the therapy's effects on bone loss which finally convinced her.

'Now I try to be a quiet disciple of HRT. It is sad to say that even feminists see menopausal women as dismal hypochondriacs. I admit that I used to feel that they had lost their self-respect, let themselves go – nothing that diet and jogging wouldn't put right. Now I realize how frail women are, at the mercy of an indifferent medical system.'

After ten years of rather erratic periods, which she put down to her workaholic lifestyle and its relative celibacy, she found that her memory was failing badly even on simple things like familiar telephone numbers. She was also bothered by a persistently sore back. At the age of only thirty-five (she is now forty-one) and much to her surprise, her periods stopped together. At a hospital visit she was told that she was post-menopausal, her ovaries were no longer functioning.

'From that day I have felt resentful – not sad, resentful – and angry that I can't have children. My mother has not been sympathetic, of course. She always said I should have married and started a family when I was nineteen, twenty. I wasn't ready for it then, and now it's too late.'

Viv had already heard of HRT and was strongly prejudiced against it. 'My instinct was that it was completely unnatural and my friends all said it was a killer. One person I met socially – a professor of nutrition – told me that the osteoporosis was preventable by good diet – including calcium – and exercise. I had read that one in six hip fractures in women past the menopause end in death. The idea that swallowing calcium pills could put that right seemed all too simplistic. But when I first talked about HRT to the hospital consultant, I was suspicious of him as well: he seemed altogether too enthusiastic about it.

'Now I feel that every woman over forty-five should be given the option of HRT. Within a fortnight of starting treatment I felt entirely different. I have always been dedicated to my job and I know I am good at it, but my energy has trebled.'

She had been having very little sex so vaginal dryness had not troubled her unduly, but she soon realized that she was lubricating again and despite her 'who needs them' attitude, was interested in men.

'My sex life now is a real pleasure. I orgasm very easily and I think I'm more affectionate. For a while I lost all my confidence . . . I felt my body had let me down, betrayed me. It took me three months of close friendship before I could even accept the idea of intercourse.

'I am not sexually aggressive any more, and although I want and need sex I find I'm reserved and modest. I am . . . I never thought I would say this . . . more feminine and more vulnerable.'

Angela Blythe

Angela Blythe is a senior nursing officer and it was a chance professional visit to King's College Hospital which put her in touch with their work on Hormone Replacement Therapy.

For nearly a year she had had to live through almost unendurable hot sweats, which had started about the time of her forty-seventh birthday. After hearing of HRT she visited her own GP and asked him about the possibility of the treatment for herself. He flatly refused, and would not discuss it beyond saying that it had grave side-effects and can cause cancer.

Life went from bad to worse. 'I was scarcely sleeping,' she says, 'endlessly tired, hostile and aggressive. I sweated and smelt awful. My daughter pointed out that my ears actually went scarlet. She was the one who insisted that I pester my GP – my whole family had had enough of me.

'Looking back, I am ashamed at how horrible I was and as a nurse how incompetent I was. I was just not coping with my job. I was feeling so bad that I had a shower put in on the ground floor at home as I could not force myself to crawl upstairs. I know that to my doctor I was another dismal, dreary, middle-aged neurotic – I can see that – but I had turned to him in deep distress and he offered me sleeping pills and some platitudes about God's design for my body.

'In the end he seemed relieved that King's would allow him to wash his hands of me. He had never really listened; just a coward with no real commitment. I feel I was harshly done by and I'm a nurse which makes me a bit of an insider. Others must have even rougher treatment.'

At King's they told Angela that she was producing little natural hormone and started treatment. 'The result was faster and more exhilarating than anything I had thought possible. I can't overstate the transformation. After four days of HRT I felt thirty years younger. The sweating did continue but more oestrogen sorted that out. Now I bleed every twenty-eight days but I can almost say I do so with pleasure. Instantly I felt younger and my spirits bucked up. My husband was astonished; I was seeking affection and sexual attention again. We had been under a lot of strain – he had taken my rejection of him as hostility and resentment when it was a mixture of fear and pain.

'My periods weren't painful any more and my vagina lubricates properly: before it was dry and sore. My skin, hair and nails all improved and if this is a vanity, is that such a bad thing? My slight disappointment is my memory. I had hoped it would improve but it shows no signs of doing so.

'My sons confided in me that I was worth knowing again. They are twenty and twenty-three and had swung between regarding me as a pitiable old lady – I am not yet sixty – and an out-and-out bitch. Now they say I am quite good company! Perhaps doctors prefer to ignore these social, intangible benefits because they are impossible to measure and put on file. But these are the ones for which I am most grateful and which are the most striking.

'Looking into the future, of course I hope that my skeleton will keep fitter and stronger but even if the osteoporosis benefits are proved wrong for me, I'm still ten times happier than I was. I reckon seventy-five per cent of women get symptoms and about two per cent get treatment. I count myself fortunate.'

Angela Blythe feels so strongly about this that she is now thinking of going home to the West Indies to open a clinic in Trinidad.

Quick checks

Breasts

LEARN TO EXAMINE your breasts yourself every month for lumps (see pages 139–40 for how to do it). Mammograms are increasingly being recommended every three years for *all* women over fifty, not just those who take HRT.

Cancer

Doctors may be wary of giving HRT to women with a family history of breast cancer, although there is no clear evidence of increased risk. Women who have had breast lumps removed surgically before the age of fifty may be at increased risk if they take HRT after the menopause. But no conclusive evidence exists which proves that five years of oestrogens taken with progesterone *causes* cancer.

Women who have had cervical cancer (cancer of the neck of the womb) may take HRT.

Women who have had cancer of the womb lining (endometrial cancer) are probably better advised to avoid HRT because oestrogen can stimulate the growth of these cancers.

Very rarely, these women can take HRT under specialist guidance.

Osteoporosis

Bone-thinning – osteoporosis – and hardening of the arteries are prevented if HRT is taken soon after the menopause. Even when these diseases are established, it may retard further progress of these problems.

Periods

Eighty-five per cent of women on combined HRT will have a light monthly bleed. Absence of this bleed is not abnormal. Unusually heavy bleeding at the right time or any bleeding at the wrong time in the cycle should be reported to your doctor.

Pregnancy

The menopause is the actual end of your fertile years. Once you have had your final period pregnancy is impossible. However, towards the end of fertility the menstrual cycle may become irregular and you may not be absolutely certain that you have finished with your periods. For this reason, as a safeguard, you should continue to take contraceptive precautions for a year after your last period.

Women over forty are usually discouraged from taking the contraceptive pill because the higher dosage of oestrogen/progesterone may increase the risk of thrombosis and heart disease in older women. The best plan is to discuss suitable methods with a Family Planning Clinic or your doctor.

Pre-HRT checks

Breast and pelvic examinations and weight and blood pressure measurements are usually carried out before HRT is prescribed.

Safety checks

Make sure your treatment is monitored every six months to begin with; then every twelve. Health checks generally are a good idea anyway, and women over fifty should have a cervical smear every three to five years.

Sex

After the menopause there is no reason to stop making love. But without HRT intercourse usually becomes more difficult, sometimes downright painful, as the vagina atrophies. This symptom can be reversed even if HRT is started some time after the menopause.

Smoking

Heavy smokers can take HRT as, unlike the contraceptive pill, HRT has little, if any, effect upon blood clotting and is not known to cause thrombosis.

Thrombosis

There is no evidence that HRT causes thrombosis. Indeed some studies report HRT protects against blood clots.

Weight gain

Weight gain is not associated with HRT. In one control test women given chalk tablets gained more weight than women taking HRT.

Oestrogen overdosing (taking HRT too early, or too much) may, however, cause fluid retention and other symptoms, such as breast tenderness.

How to do the breast test

REGULARLY LOOKING AT and feeling your breasts, preferably on the same day each month after the period, could allay any anxieties you might have. Look for any changes in the size and shape; unusual swelling or dimpling of the skin, any difference in the position of the nipples and, of course, a lump. If you have any doubts, consult your doctor immediately. Any discharge from the nipples should be reported to your doctor.

Stand in front of a mirror with your arms by your side, look at the normal position of your breasts (picture A).

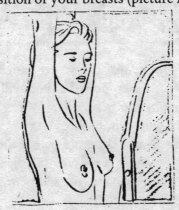

A

Now raise your arms above your head, and look at each breast, turning from side to side.

Then place your hands on your hips and, turning from side to side, look again. The importance of looking is to note the position and texture of your breasts and determine what, for you, is normal.

Next, lie down flat with a folded towel or pillow placed under your shoulders (to both support and slightly arch your back) and raise the arm nearest the breast to be examined above the head. Relax, and using the flat of the opposite hand, slowly feel around the nipple in a spiral movement (picture B).

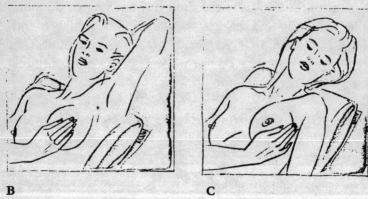

B   **C**

It important to note that breasts are naturally lumpy and it is by regular examination only that you will learn the natural condition of your breasts.

Finally, lower your arm to lie by your side, and repeat the spiral movement around the outer part of the breast, with the flat of the hand, finishing at the tail of the armpit (picture C).

Some women might like to use soapy fingers (in the bath) or a cream for extra sensitivity.

Useful addresses and telephone numbers

THE AMARANT TRUST
Head Office: 80 Lambeth Road, London SE1 7PW, 01-928 5633
Membership Department: 16–24 Lonsdale Road, London NW6 6RD

Telephone information lines

0836 400 190	Introduction and description of other lines
191	HRT – what is it and is it safe?
192	When should I start, and how long should I stay on it?
193	Is it for everyone? (Contra-indications)
194	What are the possible side-effects?
195	How do I take it?
196	Where can I get it?
197	What checks and tests do I need before and whilst taking it?
198	What can it do for me? Short-term benefits
199	Osteoporosis and long-term benefits explained

These lines have been devised and recorded by specialists from King's College Hospital, London. All proceeds go towards further research into the menopause and HRT. Calls are charged at 25p a minute off peak and 38p peak.

MENOPAUSE CLINICS

The list is not exhaustive and you should anyway first try your GP. You can also contact the gynaecology department of your local hospital, Well Woman Clinic or Family Planning Clinic. NHS clinics will require a letter from your GP. Most private clinics prefer a referral letter. Some private medical insurance schemes such as BUPA and PPP will pay for private treatment but require a referral letter from your doctor. In any case, we suggest you ask about the cost when making an appointment. Members of the Amarant Trust receive regular updates on the availability of treatment throughout the country.

The Amarant Centre   Charge made
80 Lambeth Road
LONDON SE1 7PW   01-928 6997/8

Dr Rowena Corlett   Charge made
Fairfield's Clinic
Fairfield Road
BASINGSTOKE
Hampshire RG21 3DR   0256 26980

Mr John McQueen   NHS
Beckenham Hospital
379 Croydon Road
BECKENHAM
Kent BR3 30L   01 650 0125

Dr Gillian Stuart   NHS and Private
Women's Hospital
Queen Elizabeth Medical Centre
BIRMINGHAM B15 2TG   021 472 1377

Dr Gillian Stuart   NHS
Birmingham & Midland Hospital for
  Women
Showall Green Lane
Sparkhill
BIRMINGHAM B11   021 772 1101

Mr J Jordan   Private
20 Church Road
Edgbaston
BIRMINGHAM   021 454 2345

Dr M D Gray   Private
14 St Mary's Road
Harbourne
BIRMINGHAM B17 0HA   021 427 6525

Family Planning Clinic   NHS
Morley Street
BRIGHTON
East Sussex BN2 2RA   0273 693600

Dr Ruth Coles   Charge made
Richmond Hill Clinic
25 Denmark Street
BRISTOL BS1 5SQ   0272 292183

Dr Mary Short   Charge made
IFPA
5–7 Cathal Brugha Street
DUBLIN 1   727363/727276

Dr Pauline Ryder   Charge made
Dublin Well Woman Centre
73 (Lower) Leeson Street
DUBLIN 2   610083/610086

Dryburn Hospital   NHS
North Road
DURHAM DH1 5TW   091 386 4911

Gynaecology OPD   NHS
Royal Infirmary
Lauriston Place
EDINBURGH EH3 9YW   031 229 2477

Mr Silverstone   NHS
Queen Elizabeth Hospital
GATESHEAD
Tyne and Wear   091 4878989

Dr Helen McEwan   NHS
Glasgow Royal Infirmary
Castle Street
GLASGOW G4 0SF   041 552 3535

Dr David McKay Hart   NHS
Stobhill Hospital
Balornock Road
GLASGOW G21   041 558 0111

Dr Brenda Bean   Charge made
Queensway Health Centre
HATFIELD
Herts   07072 64577

The Wycombe Clinic   Charge made
6 Harlow Road
HIGH WYCOMBE
Bucks HP13 6AA   0494 26666

Dr Wakefield
Family Planning Clinic
Duchess of Kent Maternity Wing
Hillingdon Hospital
Field Heath Road
HILLINGDON
Middlesex   0895 58191

Dr Rajappan   Charge made
c/o FPA
13a Western Road
HOVE
East Sussex   0273 774075

Dr D Miles   NHS
Airedale General Hospital
Steeton
KEIGHLEY
West Yorkshire BD20 6TD   0535 52511 x442

Dr Mary Jones   NHS
Clarendon Wing
Leeds General Infirmary
Belmont Grove
LEEDS LS2 9NS   0532 432799 x3886

Royal Liverpool Hospital   NHS
Prescott Street
LIVERPOOL L7 8XP   051 709 0141

Mr R G Farquharson   Private
31 Rodney Street
LIVERPOOL L1 9EH   051 709 8522

Dr Francis   Private
25 Britannia Pavillion
Albert Dock
LIVERPOOL 3   051 709 3998

Mrs T R Varma   NHS
Consultant Gynaecologist
St George's Medical School & Hospital
Blackshaw Road
LONDON SW17   01-672 1255 x55960/1

Mr John Studd   Private
120 Harley Street
LONDON W1N 1AG   01-486 0497/7641

Dr Mary Griffin   NHS
PMT and Menopause Clinic
The London Hospital
Whitechapel
LONDON E1 1BB   01-377 7000 x2030

Mr John Studd   Private
Dulwich Hospital
East Dulwich Grove
LONDON SE5   01-693 9236/3377

Miss M Thom   NHS
Dept of Obstetrics & Gynaecology
Guy's Hospital
St Thomas Street
LONDON SE1   01-407 7600 x2690

Sister K Lanchester-Smith   NHS
Gynaecology Outpatient Dept
St Thomas' Hospital
Lambeth Palace Road
LONDON SE1   01-928 9292 x2533

Royal Free Hospital   NHS
Pond Street
LONDON NW3 2Q9   01-794 0500 x3858

Dr Malcolm Whitehead   NHS
Menopause Clinic
King's College Hospital
Denmark Hill
LONDON SE5 9RS   01-733 0224

Dr Malcolm Whitehead   NHS
Menopause Clinic
Queen Charlotte's Hospital
Goldhawk Road
Chiswick
LONDON W6 0X6   01-748 4666

Samaritan Hospital for Women   NHS
Marylebone Road
LONDON W1   01-402 4211

Marie Stopes   Charge made
108 Whitfield Street
LONDON W1   01-388 0662/2585

BUPA Screening Unit for Women   Private
BUPA Medical Centre
Battle Bridge House
300 Grays Inn Road
LONDON WC1X 8DU   01-837 6484 x2304

Queen Mary's Hospital   NHS
Roehampton Lane
Roehampton
LONDON SW15 5PN   01–789 6611

Endocrine & Dermatology Centre Private
140 Harley Street
LONDON W1N 1AH   01–935 2440

P Martin   NHS
Montagu Outpatients Dept
Montagu Hospital
Adwick Road
MEXBOROUGH
South Yorkshire   0709 585171 x219

Dr G Choudhury   Private
Heslemere House
68 Heslemere Avenue
MITCHAM
Surrey   . 01–648 3234

Mr P I Silverstone   Private
Nuffield Hospital
Clayton Road
Jesmond
NEWCASTLE UPON TYNE   091 281 6226

Dr Roger Francis   NHS
Dept of Medicine
Newcastle General Hospital
Westgate Road
NEWCASTLE UPON TYNE
  NE4 6BE   091 273 8811 x22675

Mr M L Fox   NHS
Gynaecology Outpatient Department
George Elliot Hospital
College Street
NUNEATON
Warwickshire   0203 384201

Mr Mander   NHS
Oldham & District General Hospital
Rochdale Road
OLDHAM
Lancashire   061 624 0420

Dr Brenda Bean   Private
Menopause Clinic
Queen Victoria Memorial Hospital
School Lane
OLD WELWYN
Herts   043871 4488

John Radcliffe Hospital   NHS
The Anderson Clinic
HEADINGTON
Oxford OX2 6HE   0865 64711 x7795

Dr Sarah Randall   NHS
The Ella Gordon Centre
East Wing
St Mary's Hospital
PORTSMOUTH   0705 866301

Mr K J Anderton   Private
The Mews
Morthenhall Lane
Morthen
ROTHERHAM S66 6JL   0709 548680

Mr Hayward   Private
The Crosby Nursing Home
207 Fordingham Road
SCUNTHORPE
South Humberside   0724 849541

Family Planning Association   Charge made
17 North Church Street
SHEFFIELD S1 2HH   0742 721191

Northern General Hospital   NHS
Gynaecology Dept
Herries Road
SHEFFIELD   0742 232323

Dr June Lawson   Charge made
Slough Family Planning Clinic
Osborne Street
SLOUGH   0753 26875

Stafford District General Hospital NHS
Weston Road
STAFFORD   0786 57731

Family Planning Clinic   Charge made
21 Dudley Road
TUNBRIDGE WELLS
Kent TN1 1LE   0892 30002

Dr Rita Harrison   Charge made
Health Centre
Bowling Green Road
WARE
Herts   0920 2388

Dr M. Monks
29 Wilson Patten Street
WARRINGTON
Cheshire WA1 1PG   0925 50705

SUPPORT GROUPS

Hysterectomy Support Group
(Ann Webb)
11 Henryson Road
LONDON SE4 1HL

Hysterectomy Support Group
(Patricia Hagger)
75 Priory Road
PETERBOROUGH PE3 6EE

Hysterectomy Support Group
(Judy Baughan)
Rivendell
Warren Way
Lower Heswall
WIRRAL L10 9HV

National Osteoporosis Society
PO Box 10
Barton Meade House
Radstock
BATH BA3 3YB   (send sae)

Women's Health & Reproductive
Rights Information Centre
52 Featherstone Street
LONDON EC1 8RT   01-251 6332

No treatments, but advisory service on medical matters for women. Maintains records of new developments. Newsletter available to subscribers.

Further reading

Health

The Health Education Council, 78 Oxford Street, London WC1 01-631 0903, publish a number of leaflets and books on health issues including smoking and alcoholic-related disease.

Our Bodies Ourselves: a Health Book for Women Angela Phillip and Jill Rakusen, Penguin Books, 1978 £8.95

Women's Cancer Book Carolyn Faulder, to be published by Virago, October 1989.

The Menopause

Life Change, Dr Barbara Evans, Pan Books, 1988, £3.99

No Change, Wendy Cooper, Arrow Books, 1983, £2.95

Oestrogen, Dr Lilia Nachtigall, Arlington Books, 1988, £4.95

The Amarant Guide to Hormone Replacement Therapy (audio cassette), Dr Malcolm Whitehead and others, The Amarant Trust, 1989, £6.99 (including postage)

Sex

Both the Family Planning Association and Relate have recommended pamphlets and books which may help with sexual problems. Send sae for lists to:

Family Planning Association, 27–35 Mortimer Street, London W1N 7RJ 01-636 7866

Relate, Herbert Gray College, Little Church Street, Rugby, Warwickshire CV21 3AP (0788) 7321

The Book of Love, Dr David Delvin, New English Library, 1975, £2.75

More Joy of Sex, Dr Alex Comfort, Quartet Books, 1977, £3.95

Sense and Nonsense About Sex, A Family Doctor booklet, The British Medical Association, BMA House, Tavistock Square, London WC1H 9JP, 95p plus postage

The Association of Sexual and Marital Therapists, PO Box 62, Sheffield S10 3TL, will provide a list of members who are experienced in treating sexual dysfunction. Therapy may be private or under the NHS.

Glossary

atrophy   Wasting, thinning (of tissue or organs)

atrophic vaginitis   Thinning and atrophy of inner lining of vagina

calcium   Lime. Calcium salts are present in bone. Essential to life

climacteric   Any critical stage in human life. The period before and after the cessation of the periods, or menopause

collagen   The fibrous supporting tissue of bone and skin

cystitis   Inflammation of the urinary bladder

endometrium   The mucous membrane which lines the uterus. It contains simple glands, like tubes, which open on to the inner surface

hormone   A chemical substance made by the ductless glands, which brings about specific changes via the bloodstream in distant cells and organs

hyperplasia   Increase in cells. Overgrowth

hysterectomy   Surgical removal of the uterus. A complete hysterectomy usually involves the removal of the ovaries as well

levonorgestrol   A progesterone

libido   Sexual desire

menopause   Final cessation of menstruation. The last period

norethisterone   A progestogen

oestradiol   A free natural oestrogen

oestriol   A free natural oestrogen

oestrogen   Female sex hormone

osteoporosis Loss of bony tissue due to lack of calcium. Skeletal atrophy. Porous condition of bone

ovary Female sex gland

ovulation Escape of egg (ovum) from ovarian follicle

peri-menopause The last few months before the final period

post-menopausal After the ovaries have stopped producing eggs and you are no longer fertile

progesterone The hormone of the corpus luteum of the ovary. Induces endometrial change after ovulation and the early changes in pregnancy

progestogen A synthetic substance possessing the same pharmacological properties as progesterone

proliferative hyperplasia Overgrowth (of endometrium)

surgical menopause An artificial menopause produced by removal of ovaries

testosterone The most potent naturally occurring androgen. Formed in testes, and adrenals and in the ovary (from the precursor androstenedione)

urethra Channel through which urine is excreted, extends from bladder to surface of the perineum

uterus Womb

vagina The genital canal from the uterus to the vulva

vaginitis Inflammation of the vagina

Index